Maggie's Woman's Book

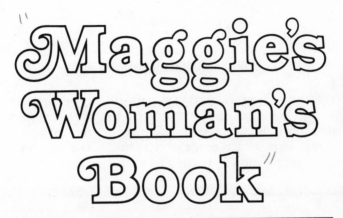

Her Personal Plan for Health
and Fitness for Women
of Every Age

Maggie Lettvin

Houghton Mifflin Company Boston

Library of Congress Cataloging in Publication Data
Lettvin, Maggie.
Maggie's woman's book.
Bibliography: p.
Includes index.
1. Women — Health and hygiene.   2. Exercise for
women.   3. Women — Diseases.   4. Generative organs,
Female — Diseases.   I. Title.
RA778.L76   613'.04244   80-13594
ISBN 0-395-29472-X
ISBN 0-395-29758-3 pbk.

Printed in the United States of America

S 10 9 8 7 6 5 4

Drawings by Ruth McCambridge
Photographs by Len Barlow
Book design by Dianne Schaefer, Designworks

This book is dedicated to my harshest critic, my
husband, Jerry, who sometimes helps me to understand why
my empirical approach works, who loves me, or good information,
enough to have long and even loud discussions over a
period of months and years.
What a Mitzvah!

Author's Note

This book contains only methods that I have found to be effective through my personal experience in working with women. My recommendations are not meant as medical advice. I deal with positions and movements of the body, but not with orthopedics. I describe the complaints of women and what betters them, but not gynecologic disease and its treatment. I suggest foods and extracts of foods, but not pharmaceuticals. The bibliography is included only as suggested reading for those who want to pursue some details. Throughout the book I emphasize repeatedly that medical doctors should be consulted about trying what I counsel. In short I only describe empirical aids to personal comfort, not alternatives to medical treatment.

Acknowledgments

I am and will remain eternally grateful to my ever cheerful and supportive colleague Suzanne Brown, who typed and retyped, ordered and reordered, and in general kept me from deciding that the oral tradition was best.

I owe much to the women I have worked with over the years who have given me the questions and responses from which this book evolved.

I appreciate greatly all those at Houghton Mifflin who help to make my books come out well, especially Frances Tenenbaum, my editor, who puts up with me and to whom I am truly grateful.

Contents

PART III   DIET

PART IV   DOCTORS AND MEDICATIONS

The Years of Our Lives

1

The Menstrual Years

Many of the conditions that we find uncomfortable during our lifetime are related to the way our entire body responds to signals, or the lack of them, from our reproductive organs.

In this book, you'll find information about — and help for — the most common conditions that affect women throughout their life. Not all women have all of these conditions; some lucky ones may have none. As you read through the first four chapters, you will occasionally find a number in a circle. Corresponding numbers at the end of each chapter will refer you to specific exercises and other remedies for those particular problems.

MENSTRUATION

Monthly bleeding from the uterus occurs in us and also in female apes and some female monkeys. After you have finished one menstrual period, you grow a new lining in the uterus. At the same time, an egg is maturing in one of your ovaries in a capsule. Between the fourteenth and twentieth day the capsule breaks, and the egg travels through a tube to the uterus. If the egg has been fertilized by a sperm, it stays in the new lining. If the egg is not fertilized, the lining of the uterus passes off as menstrual blood through the cervix and vagina. The menstrual flow usually lasts for three to seven days. This menstrual fluid is really a mixture of the lining of the uterus plus the blood caused by the lining peeling itself away plus some mucus. Now go back to the beginning of this paragraph and start over. You will repeat that cycle about 480 times unless you become pregnant or have your ovaries or uterus removed.

Menstrual Irregularity

Menstrual irregularity is the norm. If we kept calendars of time between periods, amount of flow, and premenstrual symptoms, we would soon become aware that though our overall feeling may be that our menstrual periods are very regular, in fact they are not. Other things are just more important to us, so luckily we tend to ignore anything that gives us little discomfort or that doesn't interfere with our daily routine too severely.

The obvious time to worry about irregularity is when you believe you may be pregnant and don't want to be. Your emotional upset at the prospect can be enough to make you late in beginning a period. Even if you are normally irregular, if you have been sexually active and go six to eight weeks without a period, you should test yourself with one of the home pregnancy tests. If a home pregnancy test comes out positive, double-check with a laboratory test. If you are pregnant, you want as much time as possible to weigh alternatives.

Strenuous exercises and underweight: In women who are underweight, continued heavy exercises cause menstrual periods to become delayed or to stop completely. Menstrual periods are closely related to body fat. It is therefore not surprising to find that young female dancers and some teen-age girls who participate in competitive sports have great difficulty maintaining regular periods. This may retard sexual maturity.

Gain a little weight, not in muscle but in body fat, if you wish to run or engage in other strenuous exercise; don't allow yourself to continue to have irregular periods.

Laxatives: Laxatives, even mild ones, can increase menstrual flow. If you insist on taking them, at least wait till after your menstrual period is over.

OVULATION

About fourteen days after you menstruate, you "lay an egg." One ovary or the other releases an egg, which travels to your uterus.

Some women feel a small sharp pain when the egg is released, so they can tell whether it was the right or left ovary that was active. Some feel the pain only on one side. Some feel it only occasionally, and some never feel it. Others feel all of these symptoms over a period of years. There may be a slight staining at this time; that is, a little blood may appear for one or two days. This is reasonably normal and shouldn't concern you unless you have more or longer-lasting symptoms or if you are past your menstruating years. Then, of course, see your doctor.

PREMENSTRUAL SYNDROME

Only about 40 percent of all women suffer from premenstrual syndrome. For many women, the symptoms are not serious enough to warrant the women's needing help.

But this premenstrual syndrome is the most common of endocrine disorders. In fact, suffering with premenstrual symptoms has been, in France, grounds for a legal ruling of temporary insanity in some court cases because, for those who suffer from them, the premenstrual symptoms can be very serious, interfering terribly with their lives and causing much misery. Women who suffer from premenstrual syndrome generally are very feminine in appearance, conceive easily, and sometimes keep menstruating until they are fifty or fifty-five years of age.

Symptoms begin at different times. Even before beginning menstruation, some young girls will have already experienced some symptoms. Other women have their first symptoms following childbirth. Symptoms may become more severe with each pregnancy. In one study, about 35 percent of the women had their first symptoms after they had suffered toxemia in pregnancy. Women who suffer depression after childbirth are also commonly sufferers of premenstrual syndrome before or become sufferers soon after giving birth. Age and time seem to make the premenstrual symptoms more exaggerated. They crop up over and over, until they finally appear again as menopausal symptoms.

Usually several symptoms, much like those your mother had before you, will occur anywhere from the time of ovulation to a few days into your period, when they end abruptly as the flow becomes increased.

Fluid-Holding

The premenstrual symptoms seem to happen with weight gain. Presumably because of shifting hormonal patterns, potassium is dumped from your system. With potassium levels lowered, the sodium balance encourages retention of fluids that are taken into the body. This fluid retention causes many of the premenstrual problems. It can increase the extent your belly hangs out and cause your back to ache; certainly you experience a bloated and uncomfortable feeling. Women will often put on from one to ten pounds of fluid; sometimes even more. Standing becomes very difficult for some women, as strength "seems to run out my feet."

The dumping of potassium also makes your muscles weaken, causing you to feel lethargic. The abdominal muscles in particular grow noticeably weaker. Partly this is because the muscles of the colon, which serve to move your food along, also become weaker. The colon then fills slowly and leans against the weak abdominal muscles. You don't just imagine that your belly is hanging out. It is.

Often, the heavier you are, the more you gain in the premenstrual period. Day-to-day weight changes can be dramatic — up to four-pound drops or rises. For this reason most weight-loss diets just don't work. Under conditions where you need to replace potassium and other elements, such as calcium and magnesium, you are generally led only to count calories. But the right foods that contain those elements which you need are more important than just low-calorie foods.

Fluids may be retained in any part of your body and usually will have some direct effect on your personal premenstrual symptoms.

Headache, stuffy nose, vertigo? Some of those fluids are being held in your head. Since the pulling-in of fluids occurs even in the brain tissue, the changes result in headaches, moodiness, or irritability that is often uncontrollable. Some lucky few get by without appreciable symptoms; some become deranged.

Swollen or numb feet, heavy feeling in legs, worsening of varicose veins? Fluids are being held in your legs. Bloated belly, increased sexual appetite, or sciatic pain mean you're holding fluids in belly and pelvis. Swelling in the pelvis puts extra back pressure on the veins of the legs, and varicose veins may begin or may worsen at this time. Tender or painful breasts, spontaneous bruising in the arms, swollen or numb hands — these mean the upper body is holding fluids. Recently injured parts are very susceptible to water retention and can continue to be so for months.

Lying down makes you hold fluids. Being up and around helps you lose fluids, and vigorous exercise can help you to lose large amounts of fluids in a very short period of time. *Stress* makes symptoms *worse*. Exercise relieves stress and generally relieves symptoms.[1]* (There is a low incidence of these symptoms, for instance, among professional dancers.)

Limiting fluids and salt helps somewhat. Large amounts of high-potassium foods should help much more. In countries where a very high intake of potassium is the norm, such as Japan, or among people like the Bantu in Africa, these problems do not seem to arise. You may be able to improve your health by trying to replace what potassium you lose.[2] During the premenstrual period, many women suffer an uncontrollable desire for sweets and other carbohydrates. This may be due in part to the hypoglycemia that occurs among many women at this time. At the other end of the spectrum are those who have anorexia at this time — a great loss of appetite and even an inability to keep down any food.

Spontaneous Bruising

Many of us who bruise easily will bruise even more easily during the premenstrual period. Nosebleeds are not uncommon among this group. Vitamin C with bioflavonoids and rutin, increased slowly from 500 milligrams a day (of Vitamin C) up to 2000 or 3000 milligrams per day, will prevent almost all bruising. Each of us must find her own level.

First day — 500 mgs.
Second day — 500 mgs. twice a day
Third day — 500 mgs. three times a day

See if bruising stops or is diminished over a month. When bruising stops, you should maintain this daily level to prevent more bruising.

A few women stop bruising only with 5000 to 10000 milligrams of Vitamin C with bioflavonoids daily.

If, during the time you are increasing the amount, your belly begins to rumble, drop back the amount just a little and stay at that level for a week or so. Then increase the amount more slowly from that point.

Most bruising stops well within the three gram (3000 milligram) dosage.

* Refer to the number at the end of the chapter for exercises and other means of correcting or alleviating your specific problems.

Vitamin C, bioflavonoids, and rutin help to strengthen the walls of the tiny blood vessels called capillaries.

Premenstrual Headaches

Some premenstrual headaches are a result of congestion of nasal and sinus tissue; these can often be relieved immediately, if only temporarily, by a nasal spray. Use the spray only if a headache seems imminent. This congestion is usually relieved completely by the time the flow has increased on the second or third day.

Migraines

Many women have cyclical migraines that start in childhood. Though they may have headaches at other times during the month, almost invariably a certain percentage of women will have premenstrual migraines.

You can tell this headache from others by the visual effects: bright lights or a feeling as if you've seen something out of the corner of your eye that isn't there or as if you're seeing the world through heat waves, as you do over a bonfire.

In some women these headaches are made much worse when they start taking the Pill, after they've spent some time on the Pill, or after they come off it. There are women who have had practically unremitting headaches for as long as months. Vitamin E works to relieve the pain in most of these cases.

Vitamin E: There are no known toxic effects from Vitamin E. It is important, if you are to find the level appropriate for you, to start with a small amount and work up gradually, week by week, to see what level gives you relief of some symptoms. Continue increasing the amount slowly till most or all of the symptoms disappear.

Suggested:		
1st week	50 I.U. * a day	(*no one should start*
2nd week	100 I.U. a day	*with more*)
3rd week	200 I.U. a day	
4th week	400 I.U. a day	
5th week	800 I.U. a day	
6th week	1000 I.U. a day	
7th week	1000 I.U. a day	

* I.U. stands for international unit.

If this method doesn't work, don't try pushing beyond this amount except as your doctor may advise. *Nothing* should be taken that is not absolutely necessary.

The level of Vitamin E you need may change over a period of months or years. Usually it will increase slightly till menopause, when it can decrease quite a bit. The level needed by different women may vary greatly.

Aching of Lower Abdomen and Back

All of the following remedies are known to relieve premenstrual aching. Obviously, all are ways to increase local circulation. Choose one, several, or all.

Exercise	Hot bath
Hot-water bottle	Intercourse
Peppermint tea	Massage

MENSTRUAL PAIN

Premenstrual or Menstrual Cramps

The following formula is strictly for relieving pain, not for relieving the feelings of pressure that also cause discomfort.

Stir one teaspoon of dolomite powder into a half glass of fruit juice and take it with a teaspoon of high-potency cod liver oil, preferably, or cod liver oil capsules that are equivalent to the same dosage as a teaspoon. Cod liver oil need be taken only once a day.

Dolomite is a mixture of compounds of calcium and magnesium in the two-to-one ratio in which we need them.

Take the dolomite once a day as a preventive or two to three times a day when pain occurs. Too much magnesium may give you diarrhea. Take less if this happens. Calcium will deposit in soft tissues, kidneys, and arteries only if it is not supplied to the body along with magnesium.

If pain continues, you should certainly see a doctor. If the above method dulls the pain significantly but does not stop it completely, try a little more dolomite or add to this method the circulation-increasing exercises.[3]

Menstrual Chart

Are you interested in how your problems relate to your menstrual period? Keep this chart for a few months.

Write Down: All days of period
Any days with symptoms (make new categories for other symptoms you may experience)

Symptoms: A.C. = Appetite Change   FL = Flooding, excessive
B = Bloat   bleeding
B.A. = Backache   H = Headache
BR = Breast tenderness   M = Moodiness
CL = Clotting   P = Period
CR = Cramps   W.U. = Weight up
F = Fatigue

Day	1	2	3	4	5	6	7	8	Month
1									
2									
3									
4									
5									
6									
7									
8									
9									
10									
11									
12									
13									
14									
15									
16									
17									
18									
19									
20									
21									
22									
23									
24									
25									
26									
27									
28									
29									
30									
31									

This chart is modeled after the chart by Katharina Dalton, *The Premenstrual Syndrome* (Springfield, Ill.: Charles C. Thomas, Publisher, 1964).

Instant Pain

Most of us learn quickly what we can and cannot do comfortably during our menstrual periods.

For many women any kind of a cold seat — a concrete, cold leather seat in a car, a cold toilet seat — is enough to start instant, sometimes intense, menstrual pain.

This pain can be relieved if you climb into a hot tub for fifteen minutes to an hour. Take a shower after the tub to clean yourself up. You can prevent menstrual pain sometimes by carrying a towel in your car to put over the seat (or buy a car with cloth seats), by not sitting on concrete, and by keeping your bathroom window closed and the room warm. You can buy a padded toilet seat, which warms a little more quickly than wood or plastic, or a fuzzy cover for the seat.

Preventing the discomfort makes sense and is not difficult.

Burning Pain in Side

A few women complain of a burning pain in one side or the other of the pelvic region when menstruating, usually in conjunction with an especially heavy flow.

This can be due to the blood not being able to flow quickly enough through the cervix. Instead, it sometimes backs up through the Fallopian tube and ends up in the abdominal cavity, where it may cause a local irritation and the burning pain. It may also cause (by local inflammation and swelling) a reaction from the local nerves that can give you a feeling of pain and pressure on the inside of the thigh. This pain sometimes continues for a week or more.

If you have had such a pain and if your flow is now or has been heavier for the last few periods, you can try one of two methods — or both — that seem to prevent such symptoms. One is a hot bath taken at the first sign of your period. It will start a freer flow a little sooner. This method may be messy, but it's worth it. The other method is good, hard circulation-respiration exercises.[4] Either or both of these may save you a lot of discomfort.

Backaches from Sagging Bellies

If you have had abdominal surgery, if you have not been exercising, or if in spite of exercising your belly feels bloated or looks as if it is sagging, you may get backaches, especially at night. You may find that your belly will hang out and sag on the bed. Look down at your belly as you lie on your side. If it is sagging, you may get much relief by holding a small cushion in against your belly, either with your arms or with a thigh pulled up close against the cushion. You must also try every method you can to tighten your belly muscles with exercise, diet, and posture.

ORAL CONTRACEPTIVES

All the actions of the Pill are still not completely understood. Research goes on constantly to find out more about it.

No one can tell you exactly how the Pill is going to affect you as an individual. It definitely changes your hormone system — sometimes forever.

You are the one who must decide whether you will or won't take an oral contraceptive. Certainly you first should be fully informed or should fully inform yourself about alternative methods.

The choices — the decisions — are yours to make.

The known side effects of the Pill range from the mildly annoying to the very serious. They include:

Heart attacks	Weight gain
Strokes	Painful breasts
Migraines	Varicose veins
Blood clots	Brown mask effect on face
Fluid retention	Aching chest
Increased vaginitis	Long-term or total disappearance of
Depression	menstrual periods
High cholesterol levels	Inability ever to bear children
High blood pressure	

You can get an excellent pamphlet called "Contraception: Comparing the Options" (HHS:HEW — FDA No. 78–3069) by writing to:

U.S. Department of Health and Human Services
Public Health Service
Food and Drug Administration
Office of Public Affairs
5600 Fishers Lane
Rockville, Maryland 20857

CYSTIC MASTITIS

Cystic mastitis means inflammation of cysts that may appear in the breasts. Cysts are gland sacs that have filled with fluid but cannot empty, and then grow larger as they overfill. A cyst wall is often scarred by the damage. Cysts are sometimes found in one breast; often in both. Cystic mastitis can range from barely noticeable lumpiness, just at menstrual periods, to very lumpy enlarged breasts that are terribly painful all the time (causing even more pain when you are jostled, when you are turning over in bed, when you are hugged — altogether a miserable situation). Cystic mastitis is often considered to be a "precancerous condition." Since we tend to be so frightened of the idea of breast cancer, and since many, many cases of cystic mastitis do *not* develop into cancer, what's the point of calling it a precancerous condition?

Many women have been able to rid themselves completely of all tenderness, pain, and lumps due to cystic mastitis simply by taking Vitamin E in slowly increasing amounts. For some, it takes little Vitamin E; for others, much more. As you get close to your own right level of Vitamin E, your discomfort will noticeably lessen. However, if the amount of Vitamin E is then lowered, within a few days to a week the cysts will slowly begin to become tender.

If Vitamin E is stopped completely, within a few weeks all symptoms will recur as before. Once you have found the proper level for yourself, you will need to retain the amount somewhere around that level, probably till menopause, when for some women the needed amount drops to a much lower level.[5]

EFFECTS OF GRAVITY

The effects of gravity on the body are great. If you are in an upright posture and don't move around much, there is a lowered flow of blood to the top part of the lungs and the skin of your neck, face, and scalp, since the blood tends to pool toward your feet and legs.

Tissues that are constantly dragged down by gravity and frequent impact will finally slip down permanently (for example, the kidneys of truck drivers). The only way you have to fight gravity is to tilt yourself against it. Yogis do it by standing on their heads, but few of us are going to go that far; certainly we aren't going to keep it up for a lifetime. Besides, for some people, it may not be good for the blood vessels in the head.

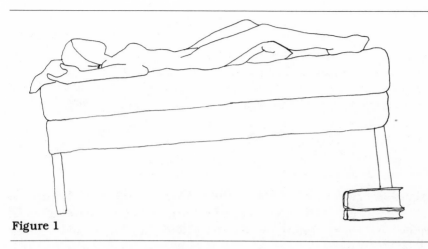

Figure 1

A very simple method of achieving the same effect, with few if any problems, is to tilt up the foot of your bed. (See Figure 1.) This position will help drain and improve varicose veins and lymphedema of the legs and get a better flow of blood to the upper lungs, neck, face, and scalp. It will help generally to reverse the downward drag of internal organs.

It will be less of a strain on the bed frame if you have some way of raising the mattress or the box spring instead of the bed itself. In any event, raise the foot up an inch or so each week until it is lifted about four to six inches.

People with heart or breathing problems or a hiatus hernia should lift their heads and shoulders as well as their feet. Be sure to discuss the matter with your doctor.

If you are overweight or pregnant, you may not be able to assume this position without feeling breathless. You may, though, be able comfortably to tilt your hips up on a pillow and place your legs up on cushions. Start with the cushions under your legs, raising your legs just an inch or two, and raise them higher night by night. But never go to the point where you feel faint, breathless, or uncomfortable. (See Figure 2.)

Figure 2

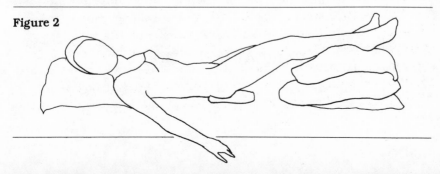

You can reverse the drag on breast tissue — after childbirth, weight loss, or time spent without wearing a brassiere — to some extent by supplying good support and spending some time in the tilted position. All skin finally loosens and will follow the pull of gravity. Look at the wrinkles on a wrinkled face to convince yourself. To prevent and reverse the drag on all skin, partly, at least, sleep with your feet up, higher than your head.

LEG CRAMPS

There are two home remedies for leg cramps. One of the best is Vitamin E. It usually takes just a little, somewhere around 100 I.U. daily, to stop leg cramps. If they don't stop completely, add another 100 I.U. a day.

Another remedy is calcium and magnesium. Most of us tend to become short of calcium and magnesium as we grow older. You can take one teaspoon of dolomite powder stirred into a glass of juice at bedtime. In order to absorb it better, take a teaspoon of high-potency cod liver oil after the dolomite powder.

If you get leg cramps, you can also do exercises for more immediate relief.[6]

URINARY TRACT INFECTIONS

Women who have recurring urinary tract infections throughout their lives know that the pain and the feeling that they have to urinate constantly can interfere seriously with their moving around to do their normal daily tasks.

You can often overcome the infection rapidly with a formula that has come down through at least three generations, passed from mother to daughter. It is simple, and it usually works. The cure is a glass of cranberry juice taken every hour, eight times a day. Usually the infection begins to improve within the first day. Taking the juice for three to five days should clear the infection completely. If it gets worse rather than better, be sure to see your doctor.

VAGINAL INFECTIONS

Vaginal infections are very common among women. Many inexperienced women are scared half out of their wits, thinking, "You really can get it from toilet seats."

Yeast infections begin easily when the acid balance of the vagina is upset. Vaginal sprays and douches can upset the balance either by adding substances foreign to the vagina or just by keeping it too clean — by removing needed substances. Most douching changes the important acid balance of the vagina. Bubble baths with detergents in them or detergent soaps ruin the natural balance of the vagina by overcleaning. These changes can be the beginning of long-lasting infections, not just for women but for little girls. It is easier, of course, not to use any of these products. If you do, by chance, get an infection, it is usually very easy to clear it up. If your infection does not appear to be clearing up at all after three days, be sure to visit your doctor.

Most vaginal infections are stopped within one to three days by the use of a very simple formula. Take half a cup of warm water and add to it one teaspoon of white vinegar. Wet a small wad of sterile cotton in the solution and insert it into the vagina. Remove it before you urinate, and change it for a fresh vinegar-and-water–soaked piece of cotton after you urinate. Be sure to start using the cotton rinsed in vinegar and water the minute you know you have an infection. Use it day and night, changing to a fresh piece of soaked cotton just before going to bed and first thing on rising. Cotton left in too *long* can cause its *own* problems.

Don't lose track of the cotton! And wash your hands well both before and after handling it.

Vaginal Infections and Antibiotics

If you are on antibiotics, you may end up with either vaginitis or bowel or colon problems, such as spastic colon or spastic anus, piles, or diarrhea. You can replace the useful flora that have been killed off by the antibiotics by eating one or two cups of yogurt every day for a week or two. And you can relieve the immediate discomfort of itching by washing well and applying Vitamin E from a freshly opened capsule.

A Clean Crotch

The flow of mucous fluids from the vagina can be light or heavy. The fluids change in consistency and makeup according to the time of the month, our state of sexual arousal, the condition of our health, and our age.

It is often when our health is poor, when we have picked up an infection or disease, or when the fluids are stale that the odor may be unpleasant.

Many women will find that the healthy fluids leaving the vagina may also cause severe itching and can eat away the crotch of your underpants. This most probably means you have a healthy acid balance at that time. There may also be occurrences of burning after intercourse.

The burning and itching in the crotch can be alleviated by a thorough washing of all affected surfaces and an application of Vitamin E from a newly opened capsule.

The cleaning of the pelvic area at all times can be extremely simple. Many of us were taught during childbearing to use a small container of warm water and a piece of cotton to wash the whole area after passing water. You should work forward from the area just behind the vagina, pouring clean water slowly as you work, and being sure to wash the inner thighs high up. Then leave that area completely and work backward from behind the vagina. Use two paper towels to dry yourself, following the same procedure you did for washing. If you tend to have a heavy flow of fluids, you can insert a small piece of sterile absorbent cotton just inside the vagina. It sure saves on underpants. Remove the cotton each time you urinate and replace it with a clean piece. Don't use the cotton at night.

Nylon Panties

Nylon panties do not absorb fluids, do not let enough air through, and tend to cause itching. You may find that your bottom will break out more when you wear any synthetic fibers. Those of us who tend to get vaginal infections generally will have more and worse infections when we use panties of fibers other than cotton. Buy pantyhose with a cotton crotch if you want to have fewer vaginal infections and less itching in the crotch area.

PAIN ON INTERCOURSE

Many women find intercourse painful. Organs that hang low into the pelvic region is one frequent cause. This can result from pregnancy, overweight, prolapsed organs, or simply the sagging of the organs from loosened connective tissues. The condition can cause so much pain on penetration that all pleasure in the act ceases.

Figure 3

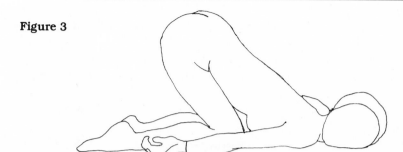

If one of the above is the reason for the pain, it can be controlled in most instances. Adopt the knee-chest position. (See Figure 3.) In this position, "blop" your belly in and out several times. After blopping, inhale, then exhale completely and pull your belly way in and up under your rib cage. Repeat the final stage as many times as you need to complete the dumping of the organs out of the lower pelvis into the abdominal region. In most cases, this will relieve all discomfort. You can try using this position for intercourse or get in the habit of keeping your bed tilted. Try daily exercises to reposition the abdominal organs; especially do the lower-diaphragm exercises to keep the "trampoline," as one doctor called it, in good condition.[7]

A dry vagina is another cause of painful intercourse. This can be relieved if you apply the contents of a cod liver oil capsule to a piece of cotton and insert the cotton into the vagina. Use it only at night to avoid getting the cod liver oil on panties and slacks. Once or twice a week will probably be often enough.

BREATHING PROBLEMS

Shortness of Breath

Many women, in fact most women, are anemic all their menstruating years. The loss of many red blood cells every month while you menstruate can be one reason for breathlessness. The red blood cells serve as little red wagons on which the oxygen is transported. If there aren't enough wagons, you cannot transport enough oxygen. When you are climbing stairs, jogging, sometimes just walking, the lack of oxygen can become apparent. Even if it is not apparent, it can seriously slow you down by making you feel weak or tired. It is important always to keep an eye on your iron intake. Use iron pots to cook in; eat liver and eggs often; take a good mineral supplement. Keep your iron level up. You'll notice the difference; you'll feel much more cheerful and energetic than you did when your iron level was low.

Anxiety and Hyperventilation

Hyperventilation and anxiety attack are the names given to a series of events that happen to some people rather regularly. Your legs, arms, or other parts of your body begin to tingle and your muscles begin to tighten. Breathing becomes deeper or faster. As a result, you blow off, or breathe out, too much carbon dioxide. You may become dizzy. If you are already very upset or apprehensive, you certainly will become more so, because these symptoms can be quite frightening.

There is a simple solution for most people. A teaspoon of powdered dolomite stirred into a half glass of orange juice will relieve the symptoms in fifteen or twenty minutes. Try to take the dolomite when you first become apprehensive or get the feeling that you are losing control, which most often precedes this state. Breathe into a paper bag for no more than a minute to slow the progression of symptoms till the dolomite takes effect. When your body is under stress, you can lose more calcium than you take in, and you may need to take more dolomite and juice. Your body will tell you it needs more by producing cramps or the feeling of anxiety. Taking this concoction every day will probably prevent your having further attacks of hyperventilation or anxiety. If you are going to take it daily, take it before retiring. At the same time, take a teaspoon of cod liver oil or, if you mind the taste, take a capsule of cod liver oil. This helps you to absorb the calcium in the dolomite better.

Hyperventilation is both an indicator and a cause of lowered blood levels of calcium and magnesium. Magnesium and calcium work best together, and the best balance of the two minerals is found in dolomite.

Antidepressants (or Help for Low Energy)

It is hard to be depressed when you are very healthy or very well exercised. An instant cure for depression is either to take a fast walk or to do some very energetic exercise; fast dancing or hard and fast sports are fine.

Brewer's yeast provides a longer cure. Start slowly with a quarter teaspoon in juice and work your way up to between one and three tablespoons a day, over one to three weeks. If you increase too fast and develop gas, go back to a smaller amount and then increase more slowly.

EXERCISES AND OTHER AIDS FOR CONDITIONS OF THE MENSTRUAL YEARS

1. Running in place   152
   Exercise bicycle   137
2. Potassium   202
3. Walking   131
   Running in place   152
   Exercise bicycle   137
4. Running in place   152
   Exercise bicycle   137
5. Vitamin E   7
6. Exercises for muscle spasms or cramps in calves   115
7. Sphincter-tightening exercise   72
   Knee-chest position   75

2

Pregnancy and Postnatal Conditioning

Of all the events in the life of a woman, having a baby is clearly the single one that causes the most dramatic changes in her body. In this chapter, which of course is not intended to be a complete discussion of childbearing, we'll look at some of these physical changes — how you can deal with the uncomfortable ones and, most important, how you can prevent problems that may start in pregnancy from becoming serious disabilities later in life. For further help with specific problems, check the circled numbers in the text against the list at the end of the chapter. You will find the appropriate exercise or other remedy.

PHYSICAL CHANGES IN PREGNANCY

Long before the uterus is anywhere near the rib cage, the rib cage will flare out. This widens the base of the upper diaphragm and allows you to breathe effectively even though the diaphragm can't move as far up and down. Exercises after childbirth will help your rib cage to regain its natural contours.

Your heart is greatly increased in efficiency. In fact, the heart rate increases safely and steadily throughout pregnancy till it is up by about fifteen more beats a minute than is normal when you are not pregnant. All this occurs while the heart is pushed upward and rotated forward. Sometimes the esophagus is indented by the heart as the diaphragm is pushed up by the uterus against the heart. You may feel that when you swallow.

Nausea in early pregnancy (a few have it all the way through pregnancy!) is thought to be caused by hormonal relaxing effects on different organs, which may be the way the body prevents the fetus from being aborted. These hormones relax not only the uterus but the bladder (you may urinate when you don't mean to), the stomach (you may throw up), and the colon (you may be constipated). The general muscular relaxation may be one factor in the development or worsening of varicose veins or the development of hemorrhoids. As your abdominal muscles weaken, your belly will certainly become hard to hold in, and your back may ache. (Urinating often, of course, can be caused partly by the enlarging uterus pressing against the bladder.) All this relaxing tissue makes you feel very tired.[1]

Part of this hormonal loosening of muscle and connective tissue affects the riding elastic sleeve through the diaphragm that tends to hold the esophagus in place. When the uterus pushes up and the stomach is too full, or even just when you're lying down, part of the stomach can ease up through the sleeve and lie on the chest side of the diaphragm. This makes it very easy for the stomach acids to back up into the esophagus, causing what we know as "heartburn." Such a condition, made worse by the uterus pushing up, can also cause shortness of breath, especially when you are sitting. The slipping of the stomach up through the sleeve is called a hiatus hernia and can result in a hard cramping pain behind the breastbone; it is often thought by the sufferer to be heart pain.[2]

The whole pelvic structure loosens in late pregnancy. It is this loosened pelvic structure, combined with the soft bones of the baby's skull, that makes normal birth possible. The retightening of the structure after childbirth is mostly hormonal, but the process can be significantly helped by hip and bottom exercises.[3]

The pressure of blood in the veins of your legs will be greatly increased during pregnancy as the uterus leans on the veins in the pelvis and obstructs the flow through them. In fact, one third of all pregnant women have pitting edema of the legs (swelling that leaves an indentation when you press the flesh with a finger). This is a sign that the return flow to the heart is partly obstructed. During pregnancy, the veins of the legs may distend to one-half again their normal dimension. There are several ways to improve circulation in your legs. Walk as much as you can. When you sit, either rock or rest with your feet higher than your hips. Several times a day, lie down with your heels higher than your heart. You may have congestion of the mucous membranes of the nose, as sometimes happens during a menstrual cycle or during sexual excitement. It may cause you to snore. You have a greatly increased blood flow, which serves to get rid of yours and your baby's excess heat. Because of this increased blood flow, women who usually have cold hands and feet may get some relief for the first time.

The weight of the baby on the major vein along your back can prevent blood from returning to the heart properly. If you get dizzy when you lie on your back during pregnancy, you can immediately relieve the dizziness by lying on your side.

Balance and weight are changing daily, even minute to minute, as the baby begins to move. In most cases, you can learn to accommodate, to feel graceful and comfortable rather than awkward and clumsy, if you keep moving.

During pregnancy the uterus grows in weight from a little less than two ounces to more than two and a half pounds. It's almost pure contractile tissue. You can actually go to sleep during labor and your uterus will contract and deliver the baby itself.

During these months, the breasts can gain around half a pound each. It is important to support the weight and free up the circulation with a bra that is large enough and designed properly. You will store about eight more pounds of fat throughout the rest of your body to help you with lactation. There is some evidence that without that fat deposit you may lose calcium from your bones when your child nurses.

In later pregnancy your belly button does seem to turn almost inside out or disappear. Perfectly natural, though a little worrisome if you don't know to expect it.

Only an extremely small percentage of women have troubles in childbirth. But it is smart to have a person of some successful and varied childbirth experience to help you to deliver your child. The majority of mothers in the world are still *not* delivered in hospitals. If you have doubts, by all means err on the side of caution.

WEIGHT GAIN

A myth of pregnancy is that of "normal" weight gain. Some women actually lose weight in pregnancy and still have normal babies, and others have normal babies after gaining up to sixty pounds. Sixty pounds, though, will seriously stretch your skin. An excellent diet can keep your baby healthy while you lose weight.

Dieting just for the sake of losing weight can definitely weaken the fetus. On the other hand, if you diet to improve your health as you also lose weight, you can actually improve the health of the fetus. Most pregnant women have cravings for everything from fruit, nuts, pickles, all the way to coal, dirt, and toothpaste! Try to keep to the fruit and nuts. If you do get cravings for weird things, tell your doctor. You may have a mineral deficiency that can be corrected easily.

Now about iron! There seems to be a common form of anemia during pregnancy that most often occurs in the seventh month. If iron supplements make you ill, what's wrong with eating liver and eggs? African Bantu women who regularly have a very high intake of iron in their natural diet never suffer from this anemia.

In general, early in pregnancy you will have an increased hunger and an even more increased thirst. Your threshold for taste is raised in pregnancy. That means you may want spicier foods, but spicy foods will add to your discomfort if you have a hiatus hernia.

Stretch Marks

Not all women get stretch marks. Stretch marks happen to some women only during labor. Some of the layers deep in your skin are stretched so far that the fibers sort of tear apart, like a run in a stocking, leaving a kind of valley beneath the outer layer of skin, which is red and itchy. As your weight returns to normal, the lines will lose their redness, though they will never disappear. Some people — men as well as women! — will get stretch marks simply from being overweight, and some will get them from too-tight clothes, which pull at the skin.

You can prevent them in many cases by keeping your weight down, by not wearing tight clothing, and by strengthening the lower belly muscles and the hip muscles to readjust and support the weight of a pregnancy.

POSTNATAL CONDITIONING

Delivery is a long, hard, hot job. You should expect to be very thirsty and very tired after you have delivered your baby. You will want lots of fluids and rest. Many women start their "after the baby" exercise routine the same day the baby is born. That is fine if there have been no complications and as long as you are careful to begin slowly and continue to build slowly.

Most women at delivery lose an average of twelve pounds — but what does average mean? We are, each of us, unique. You will lose all the weight that was the baby, the placenta, and the other tissues and waters that are involved in the birth, and then maybe a couple more of your own pounds through perspiration. A lot of other fluids that the body picks up in different parts — arms, legs, hips — throughout pregnancy, and the extra muscular tissue from the uterus, will be lost over a period of somewhere around eight weeks. That's just for the fluids and muscular tissue. Extra fat will be lost during lactation.

But the extra weight you put on that had nothing to do with the pregnancy will take you as long to take off now as it would at any other time. Unless you have gained an excessive amount of weight, if you eat well (good food, not fattening food) and exercise, your loose abdominal skin will, in almost every case, pull back flat again.

The uterus, right after delivery, will weigh about two pounds, two ounces. Within the first week after delivery, you will lose close to one pound of that. The uterus goes on contracting after delivery. Though this is a natural action, it may be rather uncomfortable for first-time mothers or nursing mothers, but it usually lasts only for the first one to three days after delivery. The contractions probably prevent hemorrhaging from the uterus while it heals itself.

Right after delivery your uterus will be the distance of several fingers below your navel; twenty-four hours later it relaxes a little and may be a little above your navel. There will be some bleeding as the inside surface of the uterus heals where tissues were attached. This will slow down and finally disappear at around four and a half months after delivery.

Some women develop clots. If the blood is kept circulating freely, if the muscles are kept moving enough to pump the blood back to the heart and are in good enough condition to keep the blood from pooling anywhere, there is a good chance that you can prevent most circulatory problems that tend to occur at this time.[4]

Even during the first week, besides circulation exercises, try blopping your belly in and out. This will give a little local stimulation to remind your belly that it has to keep not only the food moving along, but also the blood — and that the belly muscles don't need to be that long anymore. It is also good to remind your body quickly that you want it to get back to other work.[5]

Because of slight bruising, stretching, or other injuries due to the hard work involved in the delivery, you will probably find some slight — maybe more than slight — problems with passing water for the first few days. *Get out of bed and go to the toilet* (unless your doctor forbids it for a medical reason)! Trying to use a bedpan while you are already having a problem just adds insult to injury. If you're in the hospital, nurses may come in at least a few times to ask whether you have managed to "void" yet, which adds some more psychological pressure you could well do without.

If you have practiced your sphincter-relaxing and -contracting throughout pregnancy, it may come in handy now. Even if you are having real problems passing water, at least you'll be able to remember how it feels to relax and contract, and if you begin this exercise immediately after delivery, or as soon as you feel up to it (certainly within the first day), it will really be helpful.[6]

There may be a loss of feeling through this area for a few days. If this happens to you, you may find that you are passing water and aren't even aware of it. That, too, is reasonably normal, and most often will pass in a few days. Most people find that their bowels are still a little slow at this time.

Sometimes you will find that you have developed hemorrhoids, or piles. These are painful, swollen veins that may push out from the rectum. This can happen from the terrific pressure that you exert during labor. It can happen if you don't keep your bowels moving freely with lots of roughage during your pregnancy, and if you don't exercise. Piles from chilbirth most often do go away by themselves.

Even though they may disappear, while they last piles can be painful; the burning and itching can be unbelievably uncomfortable. To relieve them, wash the area well after each bowel movement with a very mild soap and water, using soft cotton wool. Apply Vitamin E from an opened capsule to stop the itching. Get yourself into the knee-chest position until the worst of the discomfort eases. Sometimes your doctor will suggest that you ease the protruding part gently back inside. Use Vitamin E on a finger (with a short smooth nail!) to accomplish this.

Washing well with water after each bowel movement also prevents swelling and irritation. On the whole, this simple procedure will pay off quite well, because the burning and itching anus is a source of almost unbearable discomfort and personality change; it is surprising how much it can change your outlook on life.

In a number of women, childbirth and years of constipation create a bulging at the lowest part of the colon where the stool has remained when it could not be easily passed. The bulge is called a rectocele. This creates what seems to be constipation. You feel as if you need to have a bowel movement. The stool is ready to be passed, but it cannot, because of this bulge, get out through the anal sphincter. The longer it sits there, the drier it will become and the more uncomfortable it will be for you to pass it.

Many women, through word of mouth, have found a simple, effective way to deal with the problem. Using the right hand (if you're right-handed), with fingers together and covered with toilet paper, put pressure against the perineum, the area between the pubic bone and the anus. With the anal sphincter relaxed and working against this pressure, the bowels are emptied much more easily. You can have a bowel movement without elevating your blood pressure, as you might have if you tried to empty your bowels without using this method. It may also prevent the start of hemorrhoids or problems with existing hemorrhoids.

Obviously, after such a big event as giving birth to a baby, your body is going to be changing fast — back to a nonpregnant but nursing state. This calls for all kinds of hormonal changes. On the third to fifth day after delivery, there is a so-called weeping day. Though it is perfectly natural to blame your feelings in some way on your surroundings, try to remember that the reaction is caused by hormonal changes. Expect it. It is normal. Try not to let it get out of hand; try to laugh a little at your crying. These same changes, or something close to them, happen to anybody who is left suddenly babyless. Women who have miscarriages and women who have abortions go through what seems to be the same response.

NURSING

It is difficult to believe that there can be any question in anyone's mind about whether nursing your baby is better than giving it formula. Living milk made to order by nature to fit exactly your baby's needs is certainly going to be better than cooked canned milk in any case, unless, of course, either you or your baby is sick.

The "natural" approach is to nurse your child. We have not made a step forward by learning to feed our babies what is obviously artificial food for them. Most of the babies of the world are still nursed and held almost constantly by their mothers for the first few months of their life, at least. When both you and the baby are new to breast-feeding, you will probably have a few problems. Any new job or talent requires learning. Your breasts may become swollen with milk and uncomfortable. As soon as the baby learns well how to take the milk, he or she will teach your breast how much milk to make to satisfy him or her. As the baby grows and needs more milk, the baby's own special milk supply will be adjusted to meet his or her demands. Many women now contact La Leche, the group that helps nursing women to surmount the problems they may have.

Whatever you do, don't bind your breasts! This will not only break down the tissue but will also prevent proper circulation. Try three ice bags if your breasts become uncomfortable — one on the outer side of each breast and one between them. Be sure you put a piece of cloth around the ice bags to avoid injuring your skin. Application of the ice bags for twenty minutes to half an hour several times a day should help decrease circulation and the further manufacture of milk.

Nursing mothers need lots of rest, lots of protein (at least twenty extra grams per day). Even when consuming lots of calcium, up to three grams a day, the mother can still be losing some calcium from her bones as she provides calcium for the milk for the baby.

Some babies take up to an hour, sometimes more (!), to nurse. This can get pretty hair-raising if you are just sitting completely still the whole time. Also, with this much sitting, you will begin to lose both calcium and protein from your own body.

A rocking chair is really great for a nursing mother and baby; it gently keeps the circulation flowing faster than it would be if you were just sitting still and also provides the gentle rocking motions that perhaps remind the baby of his or her comfortable past.

Many more women than men suffer from a painful coccyx, or tailbone. This probably is because a woman's coccyx is more pliable than a man's. The coccyx must be movable so that at childbirth the infant's head can force its way through the birth canal. The same prebirth flexibility that allows the stretching of the coccyx also lets the muscles that are connected to it be stretched. In many cases, tightening the sphincters, as we do in cases of incontinence, is enough to prevent or relieve the painful coccyx. Practice the exercise faithfully and daily. It will probably take six to ten weeks for you to feel the results. By that time you will, in addition to relieving the pain in your tailbone, have developed a good habit that may save you problems with incontinence and prolapsed organs for the rest of your life.[7]

Though you may be unhappy with the way your body looks immediately after delivery, if you have been exercising the right way and for a half an hour or so every day during your pregnancy, and if you have been eating a really well-balanced diet, your body is probably stronger soon after delivery than it has ever been. Weight-lifting is a basic part of what you have been learning while you were pregnant. Your body, which is ordinarily one weight, has had to learn to carry itself well as its weight steadily increased. This means that right after delivery your muscles, especially because of your hard use of them during the pushing part of delivery, are stronger than they really need to be to carry your body around. Tired but strong! Isn't that a clever trick on the part of Mother Nature, to take into account that you still have to carry the baby?

Of course, your balance has changed again! Remember that the best way to get used to your changed balance is to move. Take the baby for walks, exercise in the chair while you nurse, find active things for the family to do for amusement. Don't let yourself fall into the habit of living quietly just because you have a baby. Babies learn from experiencing new sights, sounds, smells, colors, and so on. They let you know soon enough if they've had too much.

EXERCISES AND OTHER AIDS FOR CONDITIONS DURING AND AFTER PREGNANCY

1. Sphincter-tightening exercise   72
   Varicose veins   106
   Hemorrhoids   75
   Potassium   202
   Antidepressants (help for low energy)   18
2. Hiatus hernia   70
3. Bottom clencher   162
4. Varicose veins   106
5. Walking   131
   Belly bloppers   62
6. Sphincter-tightening exercises   72
7. Sphincter-tightening exercises   72

3

Menopause

The ways in which other people deal with us and the ways in which we deal with ourselves are, of necessity, changing rapidly. Women over fifty make up more than one quarter of the population of the United States. Most of us now have an average of twenty-seven years of life after menopause! There is no longer any way for us to be maintained in a nonworking, dependent condition. We must be sure we are as healthy and capable, confident and knowledgeable, as possible. Most of us will probably have to earn our keep. Menopause itself must be dealt with first. If you're lucky, you may walk through it unscathed.

But there is a span of years from the mid-forties to the mid-fifties during which many women have their most physically unstable years. The rapid changes during that time can bring about much discomfort till our changing or changed systems rebalance. This rocky period is quite different from simple aging, which produces less rapid and violent changes. The methods of dealing with slow, steady changes are, if not more effective, at least more reassuring. Drastic changes can upset all your regular methods of dealing with yourself. And the language of those who have not experienced these changes can no more describe the trouble than the language of the blind can describe what you see.

We will call the period of drastic changes "the menopause," and we will call the slower changes that we go through later "aging."

Remember, we are all different: some women stop menstruating suddenly; others have changing cycles that drag out over the years. Similarly, in menopause you may suffer from none, one, several, or almost all of the symptoms on the following pages. It seems likely that it is the rate of change of hormonal activity that produces most of the discomforting symptoms.

It should also be remembered that this is a natural change — meant to happen — and not necessarily to be fought. One adapts by relieving the symptoms but not by trying to become premenopausal. It is no longer the time for menstruation or the hormones of menstruation; that is not what the body is prepared to accept.

First, let's look at the symptoms, and then see what you can do to alleviate them.

HOT FLASHES

Of all the symptoms of menopause, hot flashes outnumber all other complaints by a wide margin. According to one survey, 75 percent of all women complain of hot flashes during menopause. Almost one fifth of the women who have hot flashes have them for more than five years. Some get flashes daily; some as often as every few hours. For almost all women, flashes are worse when they are under stress. Well over one third of all women claim acute physical discomfort, with night flashes that are accompanied by sweating — sometimes extreme.

The acute discomfort of hot flashes feels like an adrenalin rush (the feeling you get when you almost have an accident) and often it is accompanied by palpitations, faintness, shortness of breath, and insomnia. In the daytime these flashes may cause anxiety or a sudden flare of temper. You can alleviate hot flashes and a good many of the accompanying symptoms with the right amount of Vitamin E.

Although Vitamin E does not usually produce immediate or same-day relief, in most cases over a period of a few weeks, as you slowly increase the amount, your symptoms will lessen and then disappear. Be sure to take Vitamin E as suggested to find the proper amount for you. Fifty I.U. may be all you need.[1]

The less dramatic changes, such as fatigue, irritability, and depression, seem naturally to go hand in hand, since anyone who is tired will tend toward irritability — and if you are irritable often enough, you will certainly get depressed, or at least moody.

But don't let me make it sound easy. Terrible fits of depression may fall on you when there is no obvious cause. And why shouldn't you feel tired if you haven't slept? There are, however, ways to lighten your mood significantly through diet.[2]

MUSCLE WEAKNESS

In menopause, muscle weakens; there is often a diminution of muscle bulk and muscle tone. Furthermore, collagen, the strong basic material of connective tissue, tends to break down. Let's think about what those changes may affect.

Weakened muscles will certainly lead to your feeling fatigued. Hanging belly muscles will surely put an added strain on the tissue that suspends the guts, even to the point of causing backaches. The giving-way of the connective tissue can be felt by some women, because the slings of tissue that hold up the abdominal organs start to sag dramatically, giving you the appearance of having a large belly and making it difficult for you to hold your belly in, even if your muscles remain in reasonably good condition.[3]

Weak muscle tone in the bladder will lead to overfilling and incomplete emptying. The resulting irritation leads to an urge to urinate often. The muscle ring around the urethra also weakens, so often you not only don't know whether you're empty, but you don't even know whether you're urinating or not unless you look. This same weakness can cause you to leak when you cough, sneeze, laugh — sometimes to leak just on getting up from a chair or doing something else as simple. This drag can give you backaches during the day and even more often at night, when the full bladder plus the drag of tissues causes added problems, many of which can be prevented or helped.[4]

As the layers of fat between the skin and the muscle disappear, the muscles show more clearly, and skin tends to lose elasticity and to become dry and wrinkled. Ironically, at the same time as the bladder muscle relaxes, the uterus contracts down to a fraction of its former self. It may at times contract painfully during intercourse; or it may, during some of your later menstrual periods, make you feel as if you're trying to give birth to a baby. It can be quite uncomfortable and can last from a few minutes to several hours. Dolomite relieves the discomfort.

CALCIUM LOSS

Calcium loss begins around the age of forty for women and continues at the rate of about 1 percent a year. There is no evidence that menopause as such — if it can be said to occur at some specific time — increases the loss. But the changes in hormonal activity do begin around forty. Osteoporosis, the loss of bony tissue from the skeleton and most especially from the spine, may show up in the form of chronic back pain and changes of spinal curvature, like kyphosis, the weakening and rounding of the upper body.[5] In advanced osteoporosis, the femur, the large bone of the thigh, breaks easily at its "neck," close to the hip joint, and the forearms also tend to break more easily. There seems to be at the same time a loss or change in the elastic base of the bone, the matrix, into which the calcium and other minerals are deposited.

Any or all of this could be responsible for the muscle, bone, and joint aches to which menopausal women fall prey. The disordered handling of calcium may also account for muscle cramps in the lower leg, or numbness — and both be made worse by lowered circulation resulting from slack muscle. The collagen breakdown can also cause breakdown of joint tissues, which results in arthriticlike discomfort or pain.[6]

HIGH BLOOD PRESSURE

High blood pressure is quite common in women past menopause. According to one researcher, there is an acute rise in blood pressure in 66 percent of women within six months to two years of their last menstrual period.

There is also evidence that the use of the contraceptive pill is involved in many instances of high blood pressure among younger women.

High blood pressure involves several factors. There is too high a volume of fluids in the circulatory system; the smallest arteries have the wrong elasticity; and the rate at which the heart is beating is too fast. Hormonal effects are involved.

The larger questions we can leave to the medical profession, but there is much that we can do for ourselves. Add even more potassium-high foods to your diet and cut down your salt intake to as little as possible to avoid retaining excess fluids. Increase exercise gradually.[7] This may, with time, change the elasticity of the smallest arteries and will also slow the heart rate. From the time you are young, keep your weight level right for your bone structure.

Many doctors still are using these methods alone to control completely many of the less complicated forms of high blood pressure.

Your doctor should be your personal guide. Even if you think you have totally abolished your blood pressure problem, a regular checkup by a doctor is of absolute importance to see that it remains low.

Self-help will remain the most important handle you have on your own blood pressure. Part of that self-help is acknowledging that you need the help of a medical professional.

DRY VAGINA

The vagina, which in youth has an irregular surface, can become smooth with age. The fluids that kept it moist now become more watery and less like mucus, and are produced in a lessened amount. The fluids also change in smell — not bad, but different. The vagina may shrink in size. This can be a blessing for those women who have had many children and whose vaginas may have become quite stretched. Now comes a strange story! If as you age you do not continue an active sex life, the vagina may become less moist, less easily lubricated, and may shrink so much that a renewal of sexual activity after long absention can cause the vagina to crack and bleed. Women who continue an active partnered sex life or who masturbate do not, in general, suffer these problems as often. For many women, however, a dry vagina is a cause of painful intercourse.

Vaginal lubricants that contain estrogen produce higher estrogen levels in the blood than do those estrogens taken by mouth. If there is a reason for you not to take estrogens by mouth, you certainly should not take them in the form of a vaginal cream. In any case, there is another way to deal with this problem.

You may counteract the thinning, shrinking, and drying of mucous membranes by applying Vitamin A and D locally to the vaginal tissue. Squeeze the contents of a cod liver oil capsule in a 5000 A–to–500 D potency onto a piece of cotton and apply it at night.

It seems reasonable to suppose that if you keep your daily intake of Vitamins A and D as it should be, your mucous membranes stand a better chance of remaining healthy. In the United States, a large percentage of us have a low intake of Vitamins A and D, especially as we age and digestion may become impaired. A good vitamin-mineral supplement is an excellent investment, but locally applied Vitamins A and D are best.

As we age, impaired digestion reduces the capacity of many of us to break down Vitamin A in the form in which it comes in fruits and vegetables. Because of this, cod liver oil remains the single best source of Vitamins A and D.

YOUR SEX LIFE

When the ovaries stop producing enough estrogens for reproduction, passions may wane for a while. As other sources of estrogen production develop more efficient ways to produce these hormones, the levels of sexual hunger begin to rise again. This period of waning passions can be so abrupt that what was once a loving, even passionate, act can become revolting or even nauseating for some women. You may want to be kind; the time will probably come again when it will be enjoyable, maybe even more so when no thought must be given to contraception, and time is not at a premium, as it is when you have growing children around you. This period of waning passion is an excellent period of your life to take stock, to look objectively at what you have accomplished alone or together with your mate. It may be a time of great disturbance if you find your marriage wanting in other respects. Don't cover up the symptoms with drugs. Be objective; learn to cope.

MEN'S ATTITUDES

Men are for the most part notoriously unsympathetic toward an uncomfortable menopause. That is easy to understand. What do they have to judge our discomfort by? Nothing shows. They have not had even the ups and downs of a simple uncomfortable menstrual period by which to judge. We should not ask the impossible.

Even some women, especially those whose menstrual periods are regular and symptom-free and whose menopauses are simple and uneventful, have little understanding of those who have the problems. Complaining will gain you nothing — unless it's a reputation for complaining, which you then have to live down when menopausal symptoms have subsided.

The best thing we can do is gather in small groups without outsiders, who will most certainly be patronizing, and get it all off our chests — sharing methods of relief, then holding in our complaints and questions and answers till the group convenes again.

EXERCISES AND OTHER AIDS FOR CONDITIONS
OF MENOPAUSE

4
Growing Older

At past fifty or menopause — whichever comes first — it's time for a fresh start. If you've had an uneventful menopause, you're all set for some good years. If your menopause was rocky, you may have some bad habits to get rid of. It pays really to work hard at setting up a positive program for yourself. If you did hit rock bottom and need help to pull yourself together, join exercise classes or discussion groups right away. Don't throw good times away by putting off a new beginning.

Those twenty-seven years, more or less, can be good years if we take care of ourselves well. Even though our incomes almost invariably will have declined, it is a fact that most of us thrive on company, touching, and good times. If you thought the "golden years" meant lying back and letting others do for you, forget it. Lying back is conducive only to dying. Literally. At any time, but especially when you are older, lying down for too long a period can make your muscles weaker, your bones more brittle, and can even give you pneumonia! A good night's sleep? Fine. An afternoon's nap? Fine. But be up and active the rest of the time.

Our bodies are originally overbuilt, with many auxiliary systems to help keep us going through sicknesses, disease, and accidents. Now, because of these sicknesses, diseases, and accidents, a lot of those systems have been used up or broken down. So it is very important at this stage in our lives to do as much right for ourselves and do as little to tear ourselves down as possible.

MUSCLES AND JOINTS

Joint space becomes less and joints stiffen, so each time we rise from bed we should take a few minutes to warm up our joint fluids — just as you'd warm up your car in the winter.[1] This keeps joint spaces open and prevents the body from shrinking somewhat.

Muscle tissue tends to diminish, and what is left is weaker. We must feed ourselves well to provide fuel for the muscles and then exercise them to keep them strong. It is the pull of the muscle against the bone that helps keep the bone strong, so exercise is important for bones as well as muscles. Bone rapidly dissolves when it isn't stressed frequently, as we have learned from astronauts in orbit.

Our muscles can usually contract to only half their length. Tighten the muscle as much as you can to pull up the slack. Use light weights if you like. If the muscle is not tightened, your body loses shape because slack muscle sags. When muscle weakens and sags, bones weaken further, since it is the pull of the muscle against the bone that determines to a large extent the strength of the bone. All of this lack of muscle or weakened muscle will lead to a feeling of fatigue and, if you let yourself rest or sit around, to depression.[2]

During this last third of our life we tend not to eat as many meals as we did before. In our later years we average only two meals a day. Many of us have digestive problems starting around fifty that prevent us using what food we do take in as well as we need to in order to nourish our bodies. Lack of teeth means we chew less, and chewing less gives many older women gum troubles, dry mouths, and thick ropy mucus. Our taste buds aren't working as well, so food tastes flat. No wonder we don't feel like eating! And no wonder we get weaker. We are using up more protein than we are taking in![3]

THE EFFECTS OF LOW POTASSIUM

Sixty percent of women over sixty have low levels of potassium, and without potassium every muscle in the body weakens. Lack of potassium can break down muscle, leaving you with less muscle to work with. Belly muscles let go first. With aging, belly muscles have a more difficult job holding back the innards; with lack of exercise and a low potassium intake, tissues tend to hang out and weaken, and all your organs sag lower. Girdles are not the answer. Girdles only cause the muscles to weaken further by removing the reflex action that tightens them. But if these muscles and tissues are allowed to sag, you are bound to have a big belly and, most probably, an aching back.

If your potassium level stays low, you will suffer from an inability to flatten the belly muscles even *with* exercise. Lack of potassium can also make you constipated because it weakens even the movement of the colon. Food held too long in the colon will cause gas. It isn't difficult or expensive to take care of these problems. It does take some attention to your diet and to your exercises.[4]

A few of us can no longer tolerate too much fat in our diet; it can cause pain in the right side and under the ribs and much gas. Our diet must change to one with a lower fat intake.

THE IMPORTANCE OF KEEPING ACTIVE

Even as you pass forty, joints begin to dry and calcify, you become shorter, and as a result muscles become even more slack. The same weakening of the muscles can make you incontinent or give you a continuing urge to urinate. This, in turn, can also keep you from going out of the house often. The less you move around or go outside, the less you will want to. It is *extremely* important to keep active. If you're going to live well, you must keep active![5]

As joint space becomes less, joints will stiffen faster. Osteoporosis will cause a rounded upper back and brittle bones that break easily. Fractures are five times more common in women than in men by age seventy! Most calcium is lost at night not only because you are fasting and not replacing calcium, but because the response to gravity is lessened due to your position. Sometimes you will get numb in parts of your body or suffer from muscle spasms. Swollen ankles or feet may result from lowered circulation caused by lack of movement. None of the above has to happen. Most such symptoms can be prevented, and many can be relieved after they have begun.[6]

There is a postmenopausal rise in amounts of plasma (blood and lymph fluids) and the level of cholesterol and triglycerides, which are at times 20 percent more than premenopausal levels. This rise in plasma may partially account for weight gain in the postmenopausal period for many women and for high blood pressure. The rise in plasma and the cholesterol and triglyceride levels may be the cause of the higher incidence of coronaries. You can control those levels to some extent by reducing weight, reducing salt, increasing potassium intake, and by exercising.[7]

BALANCE AND BIFOCALS

If you stumble, run into things, miss steps, or have any other problem with walking or moving about, you will tend to move even less. As we grow older, this can be serious, because we need to walk to keep bones and muscles strong and to encourage better circulation.

If you have any problems with balance or dizziness, you can learn to overcome them or at least cope with them. If you need glasses, you may not want to use bifocals. You have to adjust to bifocals each time you go up and down stairs, curbs, or get in and out of cars. Some people's eyes do not adjust easily. If you need two pairs of glasses for distance and for close work, you may be better off getting two pairs and putting elastics on them to hang them around your neck so that you don't have to keep hunting for them. If you keep your reading glasses on out of habit, change that habit. Living in a fuzzy world causes falls. You live best in the world you see clearly. If you see close, you can read; if you see far, you can move. *You need most to move.* Make sure, if you need glasses, that your walking or distance glasses are everything they should be. Your moving is most important for keeping your bones strong, your muscles toned, and your circulation stirred. It sounds unlikely, but it's true, that you can preserve your entire body better and longer by wearing the right glasses. Your ophthalmologist can help you decide if this is the best route for you.

The Elegant Cane

There is a common syndrome among women over fifty. They sometimes fall without known provocation. Broken hips are a common result. (Maybe even a common reason?) If you've fallen once, don't take a chance on doing so again.

Much, much falling can be prevented by the use of a cane. If you have a "trick" knee, a bad hip, feet that hurt, poor balance, vertigo, get yourself an elegant cane. Don't get a utilitarian cane. Let's make the cane an object of distinction — something to be admired — beautiful enough to be an asset to your attire rather than a crutch.

(See Figure 1.) Margaret Mead used a shepherd's crook. It looked formidable.

As far as utility goes, a Rolls-Royce and a truck will both get you around, but with what a difference in style!

The idea behind a cane is to give you a tripod effect. This increases your stability by an enormous amount, helps you get up and down curbs, helps you to stand for longer periods of time, takes up to thirty-five pounds of pressure off an aching hip, knee, ankle, or foot, prevents many falls in times of sudden body failings, and is a positive help in signaling cars when you are crossing the street or applying a sharp rap to cars whose drivers do not do as directed by your cane. Used well, a cane adds a touch of class.

Buy or have made a cane of distinction. Beautiful silver-, gold-, pearl-handled canes made of handsome woods used to be common — some, as we know, hiding protection by way of a knife or gun in the shaft. Some had built-in sections for pills or papers.

There was often elegance in the way the cane was pointed and placed, in the way it was held aloft to signal cabs, warn traffic, or brandished at ruffians, in the way some were hooked over the arm

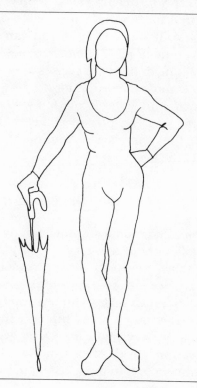

Figure 1

or tucked under the arm to free the arms for the putting on of gloves, in the way it was used to rap on a door. If it is necessary, let's at least get some pleasure from it.

BONES THAT NEED PADDING

If you have had a wasting-away of muscle and fat, as oftens happens when you grow older, the lack of padding around nerves and bones may cause you much discomfort. It is not uncommon to lose fat even from the soles of your feet. You will need, for comfort, either tennis shoes or some approximation — thick-soled, soft-soled, flat-soled shoes to pad your feet for you. Cushions on chairs will make your bottom comfortable; a padded toilet seat is a real but affordable luxury. Padded arms of chairs are much more comfortable for your arms than wood or metal ones. An overstuffed chair for all your bones is best of all. Padded tabletops are also pleasant to lean elbows on. A soft footstool to put your legs up on can help. In other words, always try to have some padding between you and concrete, metal, glass, and even wood. Don't wait; arrange your comfort for yourself. Use old blankets, towels, anything to pad under tablecloths, over chairs. When you hurt, it means your circulation is impaired. Make yourself comfortable.

WEIGHT LOSS AT EIGHTY

There seems to be a reasonably standard weight loss that occurs in or around the eighties. Since usually there are no problems involved with it, don't worry overmuch about it. Watch it closely; weigh yourself if friends say you're losing weight. Keep your protein, calcium, and potassium levels up. Be sure you get all your vitamins and minerals daily. See your doctor if other worrying symptoms present themselves.

EXERCISES AND OTHER AIDS FOR CONDITIONS OF THE OLDER YEARS

1. Joint-fluid exercises   54
2. Walking   131
   Antidepressants (help for low energy)   18

3. Protein   197
   Chewing   125
4. Potassium   202
   Belly muscle exercises   77
5. Sphincter exercise   72
6. Calcium and magnesium   205
   Kyphosis, dowager's hump, round shoulders   93
   Vitamin E   7
   Lymphedema   110
   Muscle spasms   115
7. Potassium   202
   Walking   131
   Exercise bicycle   137
   High blood pressure   32
8. Exercises for balance and dizziness   140

The Exercises

5

Mechanical Health

With any luck, your body develops in so healthy a fashion as to support the various mechanical stresses and strains to which bodies are put. With intelligence and reason you can make it do even better. A small missing muscle, a slightly misshapen bone, too little or too much tissue or fluid between the bones at a joint, a misplacement of some parts — and the body is in trouble. Slowly but inexorably the asymmetry will take its toll — unless you see the asymmetry and decide to do something about it.

There is a right way to develop each part of your body and keep it in good condition. Exercise is one way to slow down the deterioration of the body that comes with disuse and disease.

POSTURE

Good posture not only makes you look better — taller, thinner — but, even more important, the way you stand, sit, lie down, and move around can cause or prevent many of the problems that afflict women as they grow older.

Wearing shoulder bags may result in one shoulder being permanently higher than the other. Resting your weight on one hip may cause a deformation of the body in later years. Round shoulders now can end in kyphosis, a rounding of the upper back, in menopausal years if not before.

Standing with your knees locked back or wearing high heels can cause knee, hip, and lower-back problems. Standing still for long periods of time can cause varicose veins. Sleeping on your belly or flat on your back can cause low back pain. So can sitting still for long periods of time. Walking on hard surfaces, in heels, with great impact, with your back arched, all can cause problems, if not today, then in later life.

That's the bad news. The good news is that all of these problems can be prevented — and many of them can be corrected.

First, let's check your posture.

Stand facing a mirror. Place your feet directly under your hips, with your toes pointed slightly out. Your weight should be balanced evenly over the entire foot; lean a little more forward than back.

Now turn sideways. Looking in the mirror, push your knees straight back as far as possible, then unlock them and let them come forward slightly. This is a simple action that will reduce the curve in your lower back. It also encourages use of the muscles around the knee instead of putting strain on the ligaments.

Turn to face the mirror. Lift your hands out away from your thighs. Tighten your bottom and watch closely as the inches appear to move up from your thighs to your tightened and rounded bottom. The muscle you have tightened is the gluteus maximus. Women have a greater problem with outer thighs and buttocks than men do. This muscle belongs behind you. The thigh muscles are the giant springs that are meant to lift and lower you and absorb impact when you jump or run.

Turn sideways and look at yourself again. Unless you are over-weight, that tightening, made into a habit, may solve any problems you have with your hips. If buttock and thigh muscles are left loose, there is a lack of control that allows back and hip problems to occur much more easily. Chapter 10, The Lower Body, has exercises that will keep your buttocks and thighs permanently tighter.

Still standing sideways, lift your rib cage and watch your chest appear and your belly lessen. Tighten your belly across the bottom. Turn to face the mirror and try the same thing again with a measuring tape around your waist. You may lose up to two and a half inches from your waist and put it on across your chest with just this one move. Your shoulders should be relaxed and down, not up and tight and not held stiffly back. The lifted chest will bring your shoulders as far back as they should naturally be.

When your shoulders and upper back round and your ribs sink into your soft belly, it's just as if you were leaning on a balloon: whatever is inside gets pushed in whichever direction is easiest; in this case, down and out. Lifting up the rib cage gives inches more of freedom for all your organs in the belly and in the chest and pelvis. You can breathe better, your innards have working room, and your belly muscles don't have to work as hard.

Now lift your neck and head up from your body and pull your chin in, elevating it just a little, the better to balance your head over your upright neck. The neck and head leaning forward can throw your whole body out of alignment. When you turn your head from left to right, your chin should be directly over your shoulder. Check once again.

> *Feet* slightly turned out directly under hips.
> *Knees* unlocked.
> *Bottom* tightened and tucked under.
> *Lower abdomen* tightened.
> *Rib cage* lifted.
> *Shoulders* down.
> *Head* up — chin in and lifted slightly.
> Smile!

You are now in what is known as the "dressing-room mirror pose." It improves everyone's appearance and health. Turn slightly from side to side, shifting your weight from one foot to the other. Again, check all points and think about how your body feels in that position. You will feel and look so much better this way, you will want to see yourself this way always. Practice regularly and use this posture consciously till it gets to be a habit.

Scoliosis

Scoliosis is a side-to-side curve of the spine, most often starting in the upper back and most often (as you look at the back) curving to the right. It is much more common among women than men and is often a serious problem in the early teen years, during periods of rapid growth.

This curve may not be obvious for quite a while. You may notice that one shoulder is higher or one hip is higher. These are common happenings with scoliosis. If you notice either of these signs, you can easily check for scoliosis by leaning forward and putting your hands on your bent knees. If you have scoliosis, when you get in this position one side of your back will curl up higher than the other. Have someone look at your back while you're in this position.

It may take bending your elbows farther to bring a lower side-to-side curve into sight.

Use of parallel bars and trapezes, which you can find in most high schools, is best to prevent scoliosis where there is a tendency to it. What you need is extension of the spine while the body is brought to symmetrical strength.

Swimming is good. While you are swimming, the effects of gravity on your posture are lessened, and the even muscular pulls as you stroke will develop symmetrical strength in the two sides of the body.

The single best thing you can do if you have scoliosis is to sleep in the right position. When you lie down, the stress of gravity on the spine is relieved. Now you can use cushions or pillows to realign the spine. (See Figures 1 and 2.) Ease the spine, where it curves most to the side, back toward the straight position with cushions, and day by day move it even a little farther! In most cases this will prevent the curve from becoming more exaggerated.

Figure 1

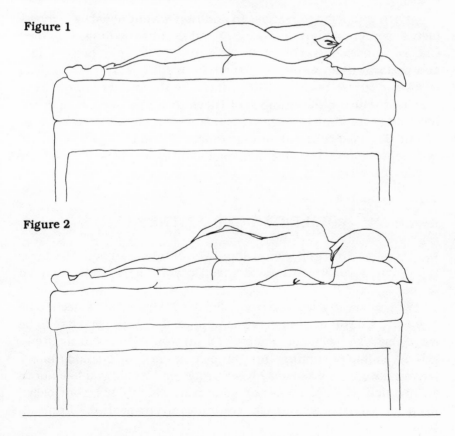

Figure 2

A MEDICAL CHECKUP BEFORE EXERCISING?

If you have reason to believe there is something physically wrong with you other than underuse, by all means see your doctor before you start an exercise program. If you have a progressive disease — for instance, a spinal fusion or spinal arthritis — then you must consult with your doctor about exercises.

In either of these instances there may be some specific exercises that you should avoid, but there are many that will still be very beneficial for you to perform daily.

But ordinarily you move about a great deal every day. Getting up, fixing your breakfast, walking to the car or public transportation, walking into the building where you work — all these little unrecorded changes you make in position from moment to moment add up to a lot of movement. Maybe on Saturdays you do a little more, what with shopping, carrying groceries, going dancing or bowling.

When you begin to exercise in addition to your usual daily movements, you must start slowly and build up little by little every day. Choose your exercises carefully according to the level of difficulty, and perform them properly; then there is little reason for medical checkups, stress tests, or EKGs. Increase the number of different exercises daily or the number of times in a slow, steady fashion, never overextending yourself. This will allow you to exercise safely in all but the most unusual circumstances. In time, as your body responds, you should be able to do more and more of the increasingly difficult exercises.

SELF-DESIGNED FITNESS

Your personal fitness program should be designed for you. What you enjoy doing, you'll continue doing. Do you like to run? Like to dance?

Where do you need to be more flexible? Where do you need to be stronger? Do you need to breathe more easily? Would you like to be less tense? To have more energy? Or are you losing your agility — actually falling or running into things that once you wouldn't have? Do you have back problems? Knee problems? Would you like not to look so flabby? Take inches off your seat, your thighs, your belly? Keep your upper back upright to improve your posture? Build up your arches?

With a little effort you can design the best exercise program for yourself. Sometimes I think (there may be a little prejudice here) that the few things you can't take care of with the right exercise, you can take care of with the right food.

You know you best. Choose first the exercise or exercises that you can see you need most. Most women need to flatten the belly, slim the hips, or tighten the backs of the upper arms. Exercise just one part of your body, if that's all you're up to in the beginning. Your energy and endurance will change for the better as you continue.

Choose a variation of the exercise that is completely within your grasp — easy, comfortable, useful. Don't do too many exercises; too many will make you stiff and discourage you. Do just a few today, and your success will help you return to do more tomorrow. What would be just too much for today should be easy for you a week later.

This is important! Always — there are no exceptions — always start below where you think you can, below your fitness level. And always advance more slowly than you think you can. This almost guarantees one successful day after another.

BREATHING WHILE EXERCISING

Muscles consume fuel to continue their work. To burn that fuel they need oxygen, which you breathe in. Among the end-products of the burning is carbon dioxide, which you breathe out. The harder you work, the more oxygen you need and the more carbon dioxide you make. That is why you pant. Your body is saying, "I have too much carbon dioxide." This panting, in turn, brings in more oxygen and gets rid of the carbon dioxide.

Obviously, it is important not to lessen the oxygen supply to your body. It is just as important to increase the supply if you can by breathing more deeply, lifting and opening the chest wider, and opening the mouth to make easy the passage of yet more air. Learning how to breathe while exercising is clearly useful. Then, as you continue to exercise, your body becomes more and more practiced at using the available oxygen; in time you will find you can move longer and faster and harder before you begin to pant.

Try never to hold your breath when exercising except where it is explicitly stated as important to the particular exercise. Your breath should continue to flow smoothly in and out with no catches in the flow, even when you are under exertion for the entire time you're moving.

Holding your breath pushes up your heart rate and your blood pressure. Keep breathing steadily.

When you find yourself breathing harder as you do an exercise, it is because your body needs more oxygen to perform that movement. Clearly, you do not want to cut off the supply. This would prevent your being able to do as many repetitions as you would otherwise be able to do and will push up your blood pressure. Keep breathing deeply. Resting after a certain number of repetitions of any exercise allows the body to recover very quickly. Slow down, doing little or nothing for anywhere from a few minutes to a few hours, if you're not in very good condition. When you're in better condition, "rest" by doing an exercise that uses an entirely different muscle group before returning to the exercise you were doing before.

Do not ever allow yourself to hold your breath during exercise. Keep breathing steadily.

INCREASING MUSCULAR WORK

Do you want a tighter body, smoother muscles? Do you remember Charles Atlas and his "dynamic tension"? Have you studied ballet? Working with muscles already under tension not only gives great control, as in ballet, but with gradually increased tension can develop muscles, just as using weights does. You need not aspire to be Atlas or Danilova, but remember that when your muscles are tighter, you are burning more calories even when you are at rest and so are less likely to put on weight.

Once you have become accustomed to each of the exercises and can do them all easily, try adding a bit of extra tension. Start by trying exercise 12 from Chapter 12, the Twenty Most Important Exercises. Then pick up a two- or three-pound can of solid food, such as dog food, in each hand. (Solid food won't shift weight end to end as you exercise.) Feel how it makes you tighten your muscles. Put the cans down, tighten up your arms, and repeat the exercise with your muscles still held tight. Try the same exercise the next week, first picking up four- or five-pound weights. After a while you won't need to pick up weights to judge how to increase the tension in your muscles. As you develop all the different parts of yourself, you will find you can tense just a little harder each time.

Now you are on your way to developing a nice tight body.

GRAVITY, THE LONG AND THE SHORT

Gravity constantly pulls down on every part of your body, compressing you toward the ground. Impact, such as you get by walking or running on hard surfaces, causes further compression. Posture plays a part also. You can lose from an inch to an inch and a half between morning and night with just ordinary activities. As you sleep, you get almost all of this height back, especially if your sleeping position is conducive to allowing the back to relax in the best position and pull fluids back into the discs between the vertebrae to replenish those fluids which have been pressed out.

Each day we may lose a tiny bit of height permanently. It is common to lose some height with time, much of it in the form of this cushioning between the vertebrae. Women start losing height more rapidly around forty. It is important to stretch the spine out well every day, preferably several times every day and as much of the night as is possible to counter this natural phenomenon of height loss. Nighttime gives added advantages because gravity doesn't pull down vertically on your body when you are lying in bed.

Sleeping in the fetal position is the perfect way to help stretch your back out well and pull the fluids back into the discs. Don't sleep on your back or your belly. (You may need to sleep on your back for a short time to get rid of round shoulders or lymphedema. See pages 93 and 99.) When your body is stretched out straight, the position of the head, or top, of the femur in the pelvic socket forces your back to arch and prevents the fullest extension of the spine.

During the day, especially early in the morning and then later in the day, try stretching or squatting while holding on to sinks or doorknobs; keep your bottom tucked under, knees bent, feet apart, and head dropped. Repeated slowly several times, these exercises can often instantly relieve back stiffness or backache.

Grass cushions your feet; concrete causes more impact. Preserve your joints; if you are going to walk or run, get on grass or soft earth wherever possible. If walking or running on grass or earth really is impossible, be sure your shoes are the softest soled and the best cushioned you can find. You may or may not have trouble today, but you are certainly doing damage. *Landing lightly positively helps!* The way you control impact does much to preserve the cushioning between the joints.

Late in pregnancy and, with some women, during every menstrual period, pelvic ligaments loosen. In delivery this allows nutation (the movement of the bony pelvis in at the top of the hips and more open at the bottom) from downward pressure. For women whose pelvic ligaments loosen during menstruation there is good reason to suspect that upward pressure on the hips, such as you get from impact, could cause the same movement of the pelvis. Think about it. Are you, in general, more flexible just before your periods? If your belly sags or if you are constipated or get premenstrual backaches, you may develop backaches when running. Wear well-cushioned flat shoes and land very lightly, on grass, if possible, if you are going to run at all.

Change While You Sleep

Your body is working twenty-four hours a day. Even while you sleep, there is construction and demolition going on, as there is in a city. There are many transportation systems running — airborne, fluid borne, solid borne — for the refuse and building materials to be transported to and fro. And, as in a city, certain rules have to be observed, or buildings crumble, streams become clogged, the airways become polluted.

Whether you spend four or eight hours a day sleeping, the time should not be wasted. You can be sure your body will be changing in the right way by sleeping in the right position in the right bed, by adjusting the air and humidity, by wearing the right clothes, and by adding necessary ingredients, like dolomite in fruit juice, just before you go to bed.

Don't waste this time. Don't ignore it. If you don't arrange your sleep positively to improve your body, your body may be actually breaking down during your sleep.

A MAINTENANCE PROGRAM

Once you're in good condition, it is very important to use a regular program to keep yourself that way. Being in good condition to handle our particular world requires very little of us, considering what the human body is capable of. That includes our ways of using our brains. We are filled with untrained possibilities, yet, in our wildest dreams, most of us do not attempt what we actually could achieve.

Here are four points to keep in mind to remain in good condition or to improve slowly over what you have accomplished up to now.

1. *Choose those exercises that you need most.*
   Look yourself over. Where does your body not shape up quite right? Where are you not strong enough? Where do you tend to weaken first? Where are you not as flexible as you'd like to be?

2. *Do each exercise every day, the best way that you can.*
   Don't just slop along with an exercise! If it's worth doing and you're going to put the time in, *do it with class!* You get out of an exercise only what you put into it.

3. *Do each exercise every day, at least as many times as you did it the day before. Add a little extra tension every day.*
   Of course, if you get sick, you should take enough time off from anything that puts a strain on you to allow your body to recover a little. Start back to any kind of physical activity slowly.

4. *Make your exercising time a habit.*
   There is no doubt that those people who have exercise scheduled into their lives at a regular time have a lot more success than those who just fit it in when they have a minute or two. Even if you do shift work, you can make it a habit to exercise just when you get up or right before going to bed. You *make* time for those things that are important!

6
Joint-Fluid Warm-Ups

All of the following gentle swinging motions prepare the body for harder exercises or weight-bearing, like walking, squatting, lifting, carrying.

Joint fluids at rest become like a rather stiff, semiset gelatin. With slight movement, such as is provided with the following exercises, the joint fluids become warmed up and are more like gelatin that has just been beaten with a fork and made fluid. The warmed-up fluid makes it easier for you to use your joints with less noise, such as you get in "cracking" knees, and with less damage to joint tissues and bone ends. The process can be compared to warming up a car before you start driving. Like a car, your body takes more time to warm up in cold weather. These joint-easing exercises are especially important in the early morning, after you have been sleeping for some period of time. They are also very important for older people; as we age, joint fluids diminish and joints become drier and stiffer.

LOW BACK, FRONT TO BACK

This exercise gives the necessary forward flexibility through the lower back and helps to warm up disc fluids.

While still in bed, remove a pillow from behind your head. With your knees bent, rock your knees up toward your shoulders. If you can rock your bottom up off the bed, slip the pillow under the lower

Figure 1

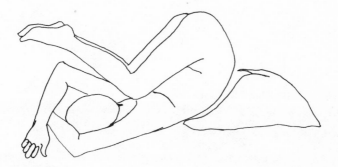

edge of your bottom, where your buttocks and thighs meet. Continue to rock your knees gently toward your shoulders. Repeat at least eight or ten times — lots more if you tend to be stiff in the morning. This exercise can also be done to advantage before regular exercises. (See Figure 1.)

LOW BACK, SIDE TO SIDE

This exercise gives side-to-side flexibility through the lower back and warms up disc fluids.

Stand with your feet directly under your hips; tuck your hips under; lean over to rest your forearms on a bureau, table, or sink. Without picking up your feet, bend first one knee and then the other (as if you're walking in place), letting your hips move with the knees. Repeat for a while. In the same position, pull one hip back toward the opposite wall as far as possible; stretch it back. Take your time.

Figure 2

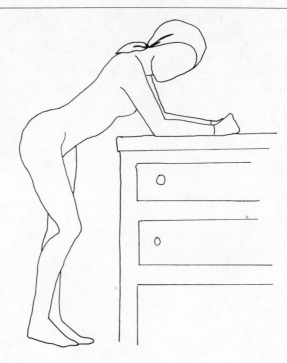

Figure 3

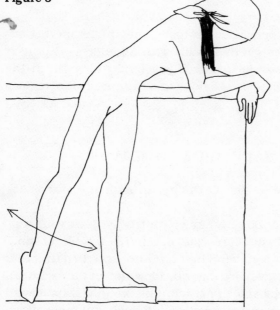

Figure 4

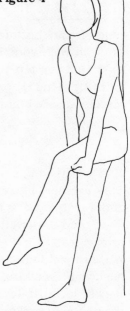

Relax, then stretch the other hip back. Repeat for one to two minutes, until the hips feel loose. (See Figure 2.)

HIP-JOINT FLEXIBILITY

Lean over to rest your hands on a tabletop. Make sure you are bent forward from the hips. (Rest your forearms on the table if you must.) Put a phone book under one foot, and, with the other leg, start a gentle swinging motion — first forward, then back. Let the leg swing itself. Then swing it in slightly across in front of the other leg and back. Let it swing naturally. (See Figure 3.) Put the phone book under the other foot, and repeat the exercise with the other leg.

KNEE-JOINT FLEXIBILITY

This exercise is for warming up knee-joint fluids and to stop cracking sounds in the knee.

Lean your back against a wall. Support one thigh in both hands. Let the rest of your leg hang; don't use your leg muscles to keep your thigh up. Now start the lower part of the leg gently swinging like a pendulum. Let it swing loosely to increase the flexibility. Use your hands to support the thigh higher as you swing the lower part, then lower the thigh a little more and swing the leg. Continue till the knee is almost straight. Do the same with the other leg.

If you have a trick knee, this exercise is extremely useful. Immediately after the knee begins to hurt, for whatever reason, lean against a wall and use this exercise, gradually lifting and lowering the knee to various heights. In many cases the slipped parts will replace themselves properly because swelling has not yet begun and there are no compressive forces to keep those parts out of place. In this way you may prevent weeks of pain. (See Figure 4.)

SHOULDER-JOINT FLEXIBILITY

Lean over a table, resting one forearm on the edge with the free arm hanging down. Let the free arm hang loosely and heavily from the socket. Start it swinging and let it swing like a pendulum. Swing your arm first forward and back a while, then in and out a while, then around in circles, first in one direction then in the other. Change arms and ease the other shoulder joint. (See Figure 5.)

UPPER BACK AND NECK

Sit in a chair. Lean back comfortably, with your hands in your lap. Let your head drop forward. Now just roll your head gently from one shoulder to the other. Don't work hard at it. Continue for eight or ten times. Do not roll your head backward. (See Figure 6.) Roll it only forward and sideways from shoulder to shoulder.

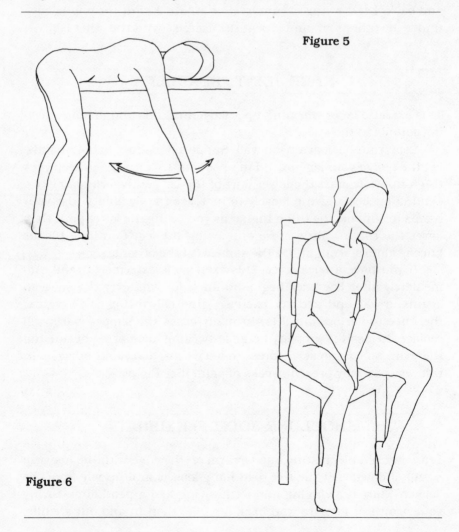

Figure 5

Figure 6

7

Packaging
Your Innards

FRONT, UPPER, AND
LOWER DIAPHRAGMS

The abdomen encloses a set of organs, each neatly wrapped separately and then contained in one big piece of elastic wrap (like several items wrapped in one piece of tissue paper). The whole bundle of organs is then packaged again by the three diaphragms, which put pressure on the organs.

When they are in good condition, all three diaphragms work to put pressure inward against the abdominal organs. This keeps the intra-abdominal pressure what it should be to encourage proper circulation of blood and lymph through the organs, to help keep attachments from lengthening, and to keep gravity from dragging the abdominal organs and muscles farther down and out. A lack of pressure from the packaging, or uneven pressure, allows the organs to slop around too much or to shift too easily as the body's position shifts. As this packaging gets stretched more and more, gravity and impact will work on whatever is loose, and organs or pieces of organs may work their way through the sphincters or weaker areas of the upper, lower, and front diaphragms. Loose packaging also allows organs to stretch down within the packaging, creating lengthened attachments. The longer those attachments are, the more the circulation that passes through them may be impaired. The blood and lymph circulation can be compared to hoses crisscrossing a lawn. If you step on them, twist them, or stretch them, they do not work properly.

A nice snug package maintains good circulation even as diaphragms and belly wall produce forces from varying angles as you breathe, defecate, and urinate.

THE FRONT DIAPHRAGM

Your rib cage and thoracic spine, your pelvis and sacral spine are the rims of two muscular bowls holding a bunch of organs, one bowl upside down over the other, both connected to the spine. Obviously, if the abdominal organs are going to stay in place and yet be able to expand and contract as your bowel or colon is filled and emptied and as you stretch over your expanding uterus when pregnant, there has to be some kind of an elastic material all the way around connecting the two bowls, especially down the front. Otherwise, your innards would find the opening when any pressure is applied and ooze out there in what is called a hernia. As a matter of fact, this is exactly what happens when a seam in the connective tissue enclosing the muscle weakens.

The muscle we are going after is called the transversus abdominus. This means "across the abdomen." It is a thin layer of strong elastic muscle set into a canvaslike sheet of connective tissue, like a wide waist-cincher (the *original* waist-cincher). (See Figure 1.) It is

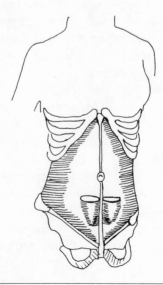

Figure 1

attached at the back to the spinal column and comes around to connect at the rib cage and pelvis with its connective tissue, then alone goes on to meet right down the middle of your belly. This also keeps it stretched wide. Otherwise, it would just roll up around your middle. The only way that you can make it shorter is to exercise it while pulling all your innards in and up, out of its way, or by using the muscle itself as it contracts to lift your innards out of the way.

When you don't use this muscle it gets weak and loose, allowing your innards to hang out on the loose muscle. Lack of use, overweight, or poor condition sometimes stretches the muscle and connective tissue so far that the weakened tissue can part. This is called a midline hernia. The midline is where the connective tissue of the muscle meets and knits itself very tightly together down your middle. A midline hernia usually forms below the navel in pregnant women, or in women with large or very weak abdomens.

If you have a midline hernia, when you do a regular situp you will see your belly come to a real peak, right down the middle. When lying down, gently put your fingers in along the midline. As you begin to lift your head you will feel first an alley down the center between your belly muscles; then the innards will push through the alley and peak as your head rises. (See Figure 2.)

If you are one of those unlucky people who already have a midline separation, or hernia, your doctor will not want you to do the exercise for this diaphragm. You can see why the shortening of the muscle would pull the two sections apart.

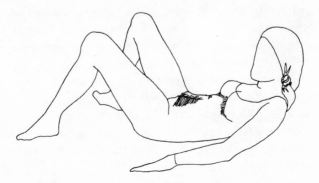

Figure 2

In that case, do not do situps or this set of exercises!
(Unless you grab the belly muscles and hold them
together as you work. Ask your doctor!)
Get your weight down and keep it down.
Go to your doctor and get mended, if possible.
Improve the quality of the food you eat to avoid becoming
constipated and to promote mending!

BELLY BLOPPERS

Before beginning this exercise, lie on your back on the floor, knees bent, feet on the floor. Let your belly bounce loosely, up and down, five or six times. Now you're ready for the exercise.

Belly bloppers increase local circulation, loosen up the contents of the abdomen, and start muscular movements of the colon, all of which makes the exercise easier.

Caution: Don't Hold Your Breath

People engaged in heavy work often make use of the transversus abdominus muscle in conjunction with the upper diaphragm to help them make a rigid base or column from which to push. The same methods are used for childbirth and defecation. When pushing, in childbirth and in defecation, you should inhale, tighten your belly, open and relax the lower diaphragm, and push while breathing freely or, at least, letting the air escape slowly as you push. A problem arises if the pressure in the chest goes up at the same time as pressure in the abdomen. Holding your breath and therefore closing the airway raises the pressure in the chest, and, reflexively the heart rate and blood pressure, which change violently not only during the increased pressure but also during the "fly-back," when the chest pressure is released. While there is the increased pressure inside the chest, blood vessels can enlarge and/or break in legs, rectum, and face, or you may force a herniation.

EXERCISE FOR THE FRONT DIAPHRAGM

Do not hold your breath if you have high blood pressure. Otherwise, hold it for just a few seconds.

Stand with your feet apart, knees bent, hands turned out and braced on your thighs, just above your knees. Curl your pelvis under. (See Figure 3.) Inhale as much as possible. Exhale completely. Pull your belly in and up under your rib cage. Hold for just a few seconds. Relax and breathe normally.

The whole muscle is shortened more if you pull your hands back against your bent knees as you pull your belly in and up.

You can pull in even more, after you've exhaled, if you close up the back of your throat to make a "kh" sound. This forces out more air and makes more room for the next step, which is pulling your belly *way* in as far as you can and *way* up underneath your rib cage. After your first effort at pulling in, pull in still more.

As you get better at this exercise, the muscle will get more and more efficient, and you will begin to see that the muscle, as it tightens further, can pull your waistline in at the back also.

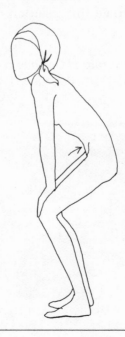

Figure 3

It takes several days to several weeks to learn to perform this exercise properly. Within six weeks you can usually take an inch to an inch and a half off your waistline by doing the exercise to the best of your ability ten times a day.

The movement, repeated and exaggerated to its extreme, will give you a really trim waistline, especially if you are carrying *no* extra fat and have *built up the other abdominal muscles.* It is impossible to do this exercise past the third or fourth month of pregnancy and more difficult with each pound of extra weight. If you have a hiatus hernia, ask your doctor's permission and, even if he or she gives it, begin very gently. It is possible, if your balance is bad, to do these exercises on all fours or lying on your back with your knees bent and your feet on the bed or floor. It is best to help shorten the muscle by tipping the bottom of your pelvis forward.

Variations

Lying-Down Version: Lie on your back, knees bent, feet on the floor or bed. (See Figure 4.) Inhale as much as possible. Exhale completely. Tighten your bottom until it lifts up off the floor to the waistline, or put a pillow at the lower edge of your bottom. Pull your belly way in and way up under your rib cage, holding your breath for just a second. Hold this position as long as possible. Relax and breath normally.

All-Fours Version: Get down on your hands and knees. With your back swayed a little, do a few belly bloppers. Inhale as much as

Figure 4

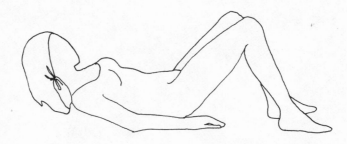

possible; exhale completely. Pull your belly in and up under your rib cage. (See Figure 5.) As you pull your head under and curl your back way up—hold. Relax and breathe normally, letting your back down, head up.

Standing Version: Legs apart, feet turned out, bottom tucked under and tightened, hang on to a sturdy support like a barre or sink and bend your knees. Inhale, exhale, and pull your belly way in and way up and under the rib cage.

After a few weeks tighten the buttocks even more and come up on your toes as you pull your belly way in and up and under your rib cage.

To do this exercise the most effective way, start with an empty belly. It ensures your being able to pull in farther. It is a good early morning exercise to do

Before you're dressed so that you can see how far in it pulls
Before you've eaten so that you can pull in farther
In front of the mirror just before you wash or apply makeup.

Don't try to hold the position at first. Repeat and repeat and repeat. Pushing down with your hands turned backward on your upper thighs helps you to pull in farther. But don't let that stop you doing it at other times when you can't get into perfect position. After a few weeks, start increasing the amount of time you hold it. Never continue to hold the position if it causes you any problems, but do continue the repetitions.

Figure 5

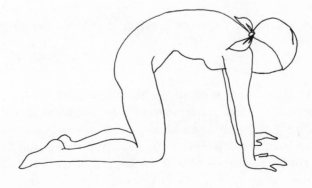

INGUINAL HERNIAS

Do you feel a weakness in your groin area, or do you bulge out there when you cough, sneeze, or lift things? Is there ever a feeling of pressure or an achy feeling on the inside front of your upper thigh?

These all may be signs of an inguinal hernia. If you have any of these signs, it is important to have yourself checked by a good doctor. If you have an inguinal hernia or even just a weakness in that area, it is also important for you to keep your bowels normal and open. Any pushing is likely to push your innards toward the weakest part of the abdominal wall. This may split weak tissues and even push some of your innards out through the opening.

If you do have one or two inguinal hernias and *if you have your doctor's permission,* any time you feel anything protruding or pushing out at this area, do the following exercise *immediately! Don't wait!*

1. Elevate your hips on a pillow (or two) that is resting against a wall.
2. Bend your knees and rest your feet on the wall (or hook your feet over a barre), head resting on the floor. (See Figure 6.)
3. Bounce your hips up several times to dump as much as you can out of the pelvic area toward the rib cage.
4. Blop your belly a few times.
5. Inhale deeply; exhale completely.
6. Pull your belly as far in and up under your rib cage as possible — and hold.
7. Gently and carefully, use your fingers to ease the soft mass back inside.

Never force it and never try to push it in if it is very hard. Let it go and breathe normally.

You may do these exercises only with your doctor's permission.

If you have succeeded in easing the hernia back in, do some belly bloppers to start more movement through the bowels, then do the breathing and pulling in and up, as in the previous exercise.

Another hint for hernia sufferers: if you're going to cough or sneeze, support yourself where the hernia is with your hands and arms. (See Figure 7.) Move fast! You could prevent the tissues from pulling farther apart.

Figure 6

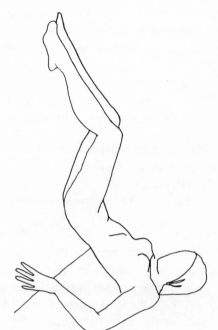

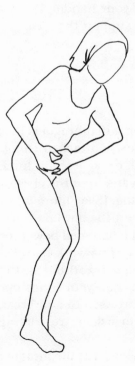

Figure 7

You can keep from getting constipated by eating enough roughage to get as much bulk as possible. But it is also important to get
the thighs up against the weak area of the abdominal wall when you
use the toilet. Put a footstool close to each side of the toilet on which
to rest your feet, or, as is done in many countries, squat on the toilet
seat if it is large enough.

Use the lower-diaphragm exercise to learn how to loosen the
anal sphincter rather than trying to force a bowel movement past a
contracted sphincter.

If you have an inguinal hernia, it is important not to hold your
breath. This increases the pressure inside the abdomen and again
will put pressure on the weakened area.

No lifting — which causes you discomfort in the weakened area
— should be attempted.

Did you say, "What *can* I do?" GET IT MENDED!

You cannot live a normal life with your innards threatening to
fall out at the least exertion. Bodies are meant to be used and must
be kept in usable condition. If you feel yourself about to cough,
sneeze, laugh, or deliver a baby, either put counterpressure with the
heel of your hand(s) in your groin, or drop into a squat to let your
thighs support the area.

THE UPPER DIAPHRAGM

The upper diaphragm is the inverted bowl of heavy connective tissue
and muscle attached along the bottom of the rib cage and to the
spine. It packages your innards from the top, separating the abdominal organs from the chest organs, and is the major muscle used in
breathing. (See Figure 8.)

When the bowl flattens, it pulls air into the chest. At the same
time, the flattened bowl presses down against your innards.

Few of us work hard enough to exercise this muscle. The shallower your breathing is, the less strong is the muscle and the less
you can pull your lungs open. As you grow older, if you move less
than you used to and breathe less deeply, the cartilage of the ribs
tends to calcify, restricting even further your ability to breathe
deeply.

To keep the diaphragm in very good condition the muscle fibers
must be shortened. Said another way, the bowl of the diaphragm

Figure 8

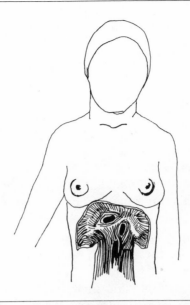

must be flattened or pulled down as far as possible. The exercise for this will also help to keep your rib cage flexible. This area of the body is almost always totally ignored. With more and more pollution and, as a corollary, more and more breathing problems, it is important to use your lungs as efficiently as possible. Women, in any case, do not have the lung capacity of men. If you ever feel short of breath on a foggy day or when going up stairs or because you have smoked, you would do well to do this exercise each morning.

EXERCISE FOR THE UPPER DIAPHRAGM

Each morning take in a little gasp of breath — mouth closed — then another, another, and keep on till you can't take any more. Then, if it doesn't make you dizzy, hold your breath as long as possible; let go when you must.

Next, in one long, large inhale, take in as much air as you possibly can, and, again, hold it as long as you can. But don't let yourself get dizzy, and don't close your mouth or throat so that the pressure inside the chest goes up.

Eight or ten repetitions of this exercise each morning should help you keep your rib cage flexible and your diaphragm strongly elastic.

HIATUS HERNIA

During pregnancy there is a loosening of the bond around the esophagus as it passes through the diaphragm. As the uterus pushes up, or when you lie down or push for a bowel movement, the stomach is pressed up against the upper diaphragm and this opening. At times, parts of the stomach are actually pushed up through, or slide through, this opening in the diaphragm and lie in the chest, resting on top of the diaphragm. The burning sensation we call heartburn occurs as stomach acids back up from that pocket of stomach into the esophagus. This opening in the diaphragm can remain stretched after pregnancy and can cause lifetime problems. Overweight women may also suffer from hiatus hernias.

These simple suggestions may relieve your symptoms and even prevent them. Certainly your problems will be reduced.

1. Eat smaller meals and increase the number of meals a day to make up necessary calories.
2. Eat only when you are calm and relaxed.
3. Eat quite a while before you lie down.
4. If you must lie down after eating, keep your head and shoulders raised.
5. Do not lean over immediately after eating. If burning or discomfort starts, stand up, lift your arms overhead, and jump or bounce up and down a few times.
6. Follow the jumping with a little milk to act as an antacid. A paste of powdered milk mixed into fluid whole milk will make a better coating of the esophagus. If you can't digest milk, chew up a couple of calcium-magnesium (dolomite) tablets or bone-meal tablets before swallowing them.
7. If you must take capsules or tablets of any kind, whether medication or vitamins, chew those that aren't too repulsive and take the others, one at a time, with yogurt, cottage cheese, or something else of that consistency. Make sure each capsule or pill is well down before you take another.

BREATHING WHEN PREGNANT OR OVERWEIGHT

It would be difficult to deny that our entire system is put together to accommodate pregnancies. Where men almost invariably use abdominal muscles to breathe, women tend to breathe mostly from the chest unless trained to do otherwise. Since, during pregnancy, it becomes more and more difficult to tighten the belly muscles to aid in breathing, this seems like a remarkably sensible system.

As the uterus slowly rises, breathing patterns have to change. Eventually, it is impossible for the upper diaphragm to flatten fully with the uterus pushing back. That is precisely why you want to strengthen that diaphragm before pregnancy.

Early on in pregnancy the lower ribs flare a little as if they expect the uterus at any moment. This gives you a thickening waistline and essentially makes the bowl of the diaphragm shallower and wider. Now when you breathe, the diaphragm can not descend as far as it did before, but that is compensated for by greater chest movement.

It's important and it really feels good to work hard at efficient chest-breathing. But chest-breathing will not work well unless the diaphragm is strong enough not to give (and rise weakly) as the chest expands. Strengthen the diaphragm by doing the breathing exercises at the beginning of the chapter. To get as much side action through the ribs as possible, feel low down on your sides over the ribs as you inhale as deeply as possible. Try to get the ribs to stretch out sideways as you inhale.

Bring your arms up and out overhead while you breathe in strongly. This opens and further lifts the rib cage, and the diaphragm with it, and helps bring in more oxygen. Feels great! — even when you're not pregnant. If you stand up to do this exercise, you will be able to breathe even more deeply. Keep your bottom tucked under as you lift your arms. Keeping your upper back muscles strong allows your chest to stay lifted up over the ascending uterus. This will keep you much more comfortable and breathing much more efficiently whether or not you're pregnant.

THE LOWER DIAPHRAGM

The upper diaphragm up over our belly helps us breathe, but we have another one, the lower diaphragm, which stretches across the pelvis. Through this sheet of muscle pass the purse-string closures and openers, the sphincters. Common to men and women are the urethral sphincter, for passing water, and the anal sphincter, for passing solids from the bowels. In the female there is also the vaginal sphincter, for sexual intercourse, for passing the uterine lining off monthly, and for giving birth.

EXERCISE FOR INCONTINENCE

If you wet yourself when you laugh or sneeze, when you exercise or jog, or just on getting out of a chair or walking — if you pass even a few drops of urine when you do not intend to — you should try to recover function to stop the leakage.

Incontinence may have a neurological basis, but you'll never know if you can stop yourself from leaking until you give it a good try.

For most people, a simple exercise is all that is needed to take care of incontinence. It can also do a lot toward helping prevent prolapse of the uterus and bladder (the falling through into the vagina of these organs); and it helps with hemorrhoids and constipation. Give the exercise at least a four-to-six-week trial to regain control. For some people it may take a little longer.

A muscle sheet called the pubo-coccygeal muscle is hung between the bone in the pubic area and the coccyx, or tailbone. (See Figure 9.) From now on, when you go to the toilet, take the time to be really conscious of how it feels when you are having a bowel movement and passing water. You are feeling the action of this muscle.

Though it is true that with time and an educated perineum you can control each of your three lower sphincters separately, such virtuosity is not only unnecessary, but for most of us, in the very beginning, literally impossible. The looseness of the muscles — their lack of education — makes it possible for you to deal with them

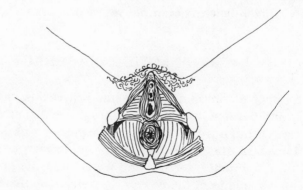

Figure 9

only in a rather gross manner. You just try to tighten them all at once. Try to stop the flow of urine. Tighten everything you can in the whole area. This gross control itself is difficult in the beginning when there is severe weakness of the muscle. In the beginning, the weakness of the sphincters may also make you feel as though you might not be able to start again once you do stop.

Many women are not aware when urine starts to flow because there is a lack of sensation. Some find that once they allow the flow of urine to begin, it is almost impossible to stop it. But take heart: when the bladder is almost empty, a certain amount of control *is* possible. At the first point that you can, stop the flow of urine. Day by day the stopping *and* starting will become more familiar and more easily reproduced. If it is difficult to start again, spread your knees apart and lean your belly in against your thighs. At the same time, push in on your lower belly with your hands. The tightening up of the sphincter can be practiced all day long no matter where you are.

Practice this exercise every time you urinate — let the flow start, then stop it again — till you can stop and start the urine at least five times. By the time you can do this, you will also have gained the strength to stop a little closer to the beginning of urination. You know you are gaining good control when you can stop the flow almost immediately after urination begins, even when you have a very full bladder.

With age, all muscle is said to become weaker; with every pregnancy, the sphincters are stretched and weakened (incontinence is greatest among women who are between thirty-five and thirty-nine); with every menstrual period, there is a loss of potassium that will cause the sphincters to be a little weaker until the potassium is replaced; with any degree of overweight or with the use of any bouncing exercises, the pressure on this area will be increased. For all these reasons it is extremely important to make this exercise of tightening the sphincter an "every time" exercise. Get yourself into the habit of doing the stopping and starting *every single time you urinate!*

LETTING DOWN

The opposite of the tightening is the loosening, which allows urination to commence, allows you to pass a bowel movement, and allows you to open the passageway through which a baby can pass. In some cases it also affords relief of painful menstruation and of hemorrhoids.

With any pain on urinating, with constipation, hemorrhoids, painful menstruation, painful intercourse, and with childbirth, there is a tension response that can cause you to tighten up when it would be much more helpful and much less painful to "let go." This exercise will help teach you how to let go on command.

Once you have regained gross control through the exercise for incontinence, the next step follows. When you start tightening, tighten more slowly and **this is important!** make the tightening as hard as you possibly can. Now do the same thing when you loosen. Loosen the sphincters slowly and keep letting the muscles get looser and looser till you begin to get a real feeling for how very far you can go in both directions: how far you can tighten them, and how completely you can loosen them.

If you are letting down the right way, each time you loosen the sphincters you should be able to release a few drops of urine. It seems rather sensible to do this exercise only when you are on the toilet unless you are practicing for childbirth, when you should do it in your childbirth position, whatever that is going to be. Remember, though, to urinate before you do the letting-down exercise in your childbirth position, since if you think you may wet your exercise mat, you are going to hold back, if only a little, and spoil the whole effect you're after — that of letting go completely.

The tightening part of the exercise can be done at any time. The release when you are off the toilet should be slow and under control and only in the rest position, that point at which you are conscious of neither tightening nor loosening. You'll find it with practice. Practice on the toilet!

Another feature of the exercise, important to many women, is the aspect of increased sexual pleasure. For some women, the exercise alone is enough to give sexual stimulation. Practicing the exercise certainly gives you better control of the muscles in this area, increases local circulation, helps to support the weight of the contents of the abdominal cavity, and in general increases local health.

A common problem with older women is the back flow of urine. The urethra, the tube through which the urine flows, becomes flabby, and some urine backs up a little into the tube. It may very well be due to relaxed muscle caused by hormonal changes induced by a lack of potassium, a condition common in older women. This dysfunction can increase the chance of urinary infections and pain, as well as the discomfort and embarrassment caused by the leaking that accompanies the infection and weakness of the urethra.

Knee-Chest Position

The pressure that comes from being overweight or from organs sagging onto the perineum can cause already weakened sphincters to gape further — even, at times, allowing the organs to sag or fall through. Older women and all women who are overweight should practice the exercise at times in the knee-chest position. This moves the weight of your innards off the perineum and allows you to tighten the sphincters more. If this position makes you dizzy or breathless, try an all-fours position. Let your head hang. When you do the exercise off the toilet, just do the part that tightens and then releases only to the rest position.

There is a tendency in all of us to forget a problem once it is taken care of. Forget this one, and the results will come back to haunt you. This is a very simple exercise; it takes no extra time and gives you many long-term benefits. Get yourself in the habit. Do it every time you urinate, every time you have a bowel movement, every time you have sexual intercourse.

In intercourse we contract our "adjustable wrench" to meet — or make — our own enjoyment. Sexual enjoyment sometimes declines with pregnancies and with age. This loss of feeling may be partially due to the poor condition of the lower diaphragm and the vaginal sphincter.

HEMORRHOIDS

If you suffer from hemorrhoids, the important part of this exercise will be the part where you learn to *loosen* the anal sphincter at will. The more completely you can train yourself to loosen the anal sphincter, the more complete your relief from pain will be.

Hemorrhoids occur when the veins at the rectum and anus become engorged with blood. They sometimes push out through the anal sphincter; then the sphincter tightens around the enlarged blood vessel, engorging it further. The pain and itching can be excruciating. A combination of the exercises above, done in the knee-chest position, will generally give much relief. Even greater relief can be had by adding to these a final bit of help. Cut or bite open the

Figure 10

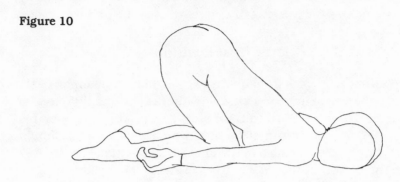

end of a capsule of Vitamin E. Put a little on a clean finger (without a long or jagged nail) and use this finger to ease as much of the hemorrhoids as you can back inside the sphincter. For reasons unknown, Vitamin E quickly and greatly relieves the itching. Getting the swollen blood vessels back inside permits the blood to flow through them. Doing the exercises in the knee-chest position allows gravity to help the blood vessels drain.

Get on your hands and knees, on the floor, your bottom up in the air. Bring your shoulders and head down to one side of the floor and put your arms along the floor by your legs. What a relief this is! (See Figure 10.)

Not now, but after you've gotten relief, practice all the sphincter exercises to the point where you can loosen the sphincter on command. Then it becomes easier to loosen it when you need to.

8

Belly Muscles

The belly muscles may well be the most difficult part of the body for women to control through the years.

Potassium-dumping before menstrual periods and during and after menopause weakens all muscle. The belly muscles, because of their length and also because of the weight of organs leaning against them, are usually hardest hit. Lack of enough protein can also weaken these muscles. Hormonal influences lower muscle and colon tone during menstrual periods and pregnancies. Pregnancy can stretch belly muscle and skin seriously. There is also diminution and weakening of muscle during and after menopause. These all can cause the belly muscles and the contents of the belly, which depend on those muscles for support, to hang down with gravity. Because the basin of the pelvis can no longer contain the mass, the belly will hang out. If the basin of the pelvis is tipped back either from poor posture, weak belly muscles, or the wearing of heels, the problems mount from simple sagging belly to aching back.

On women some hormonal fat is deposited over the belly muscles. This is normal and good, but the excessive amount of fat also is subject to gravity and adds a greater burden to posture, to belly muscles, and to skin.

Both posture and belly muscles must be in excellent condition at all times to keep you in the best condition for a lifetime. Just when they feel weakest — during and before menstrual periods, during pregnancy, in the postnatal period, when you're overweight, and when you're in or past menopause — is when you must work your belly muscles their hardest. Force on yourself correct posture; force those belly muscles to contract and to hold you. You will have positively better health for it — and what a tight belly can do for your self-confidence is amazing!

THE WAISTLINE

Making your waistline smaller gives you a great sense of accomplishment in a hurry. The muscles of the waist, which are also muscles of the abdomen, respond more rapidly to intensive exercise than many other muscles, partly because even with much work they seldom get stiff or uncomfortable.

The way your waist will look, either before or after exercise, will be totally individual because we all are built so differently. With your fingers, feel where the very lowest rib comes at the side of your waist. If the space between the rib cage and the top of your pelvis is large, there is a good chance that you can get your waistline to look very small. One and a half to two inches between the last rib and top of your pelvis is an extraordinarily large space. A very small space will make it very unlikely that you can make your waistline smaller at the sides. In that case, concentrate on the front and center so that you can develop a small waistline front to back.

If your rib cage comes down in a reasonably straight line to your waistline, it will be more difficult to achieve the look of a small waist from the front or back view, but it may look quite small from a side view. The same goes for the pelvis. If it comes up straight from the hip joint to the waist, you will want to go after the side view instead. If, on the other hand, the rib cage or the pelvis — especially both — slant in to the waist, you will look smaller through the waist from the front and back. But if you are not in good condition, this may still take some work. Fat beyond a certain small amount for padding will certainly need to be lost or worked off.

SITUPS

Read the cautions and suggestions and then, working steadily, a little more each day, begin to move forward on the variations. Begin the exercises on your bed, if you want to. Then, if it is comfortable for you, do them sitting on the floor with your back a little away from the wall. Go on to chair or wall situps.

What the Exercise Does for You

The most obvious work of this exercise is in the use of the rectus abdominus, the pair of muscles that are like straps connecting from the middle of your rib cage at the top to your pubic bone at the bottom. This pair of muscles is about three inches wide at the rib cage and has added strength by being connected over a reasonably wide area and to several ribs. The muscle is not just one long, unbroken line; above the navel there are three insertions of connective tissue, or lines, across the muscle. From the navel down there is one rather long, unbroken length of muscle that ends at the pubic bone. This portion of muscle is more difficult to get really hard and flat. There are some other methods to reach this area that we will cover later. This area in a woman tends to have a natural covering of body fat, which is difficult to get rid of without losing weight to the point of being gaunt. The little pad of fat is considered (and has been throughout history) a mark of beauty and femininity. Gauntness is not!

There is no necessity to sit on the floor. If you know that you cannot get down onto or up from the floor easily, sit on a wide bed to do the situps. If there is any danger of your losing your balance, have the sides of the bed protected so that there is something to keep you from falling to the floor.

If you prefer to exercise on the floor but have bones that hurt when you roll on them, try a thick rug or mat or a bunch of towels under you. This is such a useful exercise, it should not be discarded except for medical reasons.

Beginning Situps

If you happen to be in very poor condition, you may choose to do your beginning situps in a chair. A pillow in the chair is allowed if your bottom is bony. Sit on the outside edge of the chair with your feet on the floor. Put your chin on your chest and let your lower back sink back toward the back of the chair and, with your arms out in front of you, roll back. If you *fell* back rather than rolled back, move your bottom a little farther back in the chair. You may also need to sit slightly farther back if your feet came up off the floor. If your feet don't stay down because they don't quite touch the floor in the first place, put a cushion or a box under them — anything that will allow you to keep your feet firmly planted. As you improve, move your bottom out farther and farther toward the front edge of the chair.

Put your arms out straight in front, with your knees bent just a little. Sit as close as you need to the back of a chair, roll smoothly, not too slowly.

To do a situp on the floor (or bed), sit with your knees bent. Lean back on your elbows, get your waistline flat to the floor by moving your elbows farther apart or by tightening up your bottom, lifting it off the floor and moving it farther along toward your feet. (See Figure 1.) When your waistline is flat to the floor move your arms off the floor and hold them in front of you. Start with your head on the floor. Lift your head and tuck your chin to your chest, pursing your mouth and breathing out as you do, time after time. Then bring your shoulders up also. Continue coming up a little higher each time.

In a situp, the body should rise rolling forward first from the head, then from the shoulders. Keep rolling up, *without arching your back from the floor,* until you're just sitting on the back of your pelvis (not way forward on the tips of your bottom bone because this will arch your back). Keep your chin on your chest at all times. Keep your ribs in front as close to your hipbones as possible by curling forward. Keep your knees bent and your feet on the floor without your feet being held down by anything.

Curl back down to the chair or the floor, one vertebra at a time, keeping your chin on your chest as long as possible.

Try not to use momentum, especially when you are just beginning. The act of throwing yourself forward can be enough to give you little problems if you are not in very good condition through the neck, shoulders, upper back, and lower back.

Figure 1

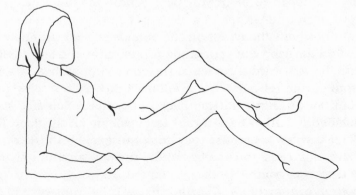

If your shoulders ache afterward, and you know of no reason why, you are probably using momentum without being aware of it. Watch yourself carefully. Make sure that there is no point in your smooth rolling-up where you suddenly jerk forward. The point where you may jerk forward is usually when your lower and upper back (almost to your shoulders) are still on the floor; this is when you are most likely to try to arch your back. Don't let that happen!

Be careful not to hold your breath. Instead, continue to breathe smoothly out as you roll up, in as you go down, because your body needs *more* oxygen when it's moving. If you catch yourself holding your breath, remember that this will not only push up your blood pressure, but will also tighten the muscles over a forced-out belly wall. Letting go little catches of breath from the back of your throat is also a mistake and will lower your intake of oxygen, interfere with your blood pressure, and make less than perfect a really useful exercise. It will also reduce the number of situps you would otherwise be able to do. Resting after a certain number of repetitions of any exercise allows the body to recover very quickly. Either rest completely, or rest by doing an exercise that uses an entirely different muscle group and then return to doing situps, or move back to an easier version instead of quitting completely.

Variations

These variations are for more difficult versions of the situp:
- Do the situps with your arms folded below your breasts.
- Bend your knees a little more, by bringing your feet closer (only if your feet don't come up off the floor when you exercise).
- Place your hands behind your head and *your elbows forward.* Don't jerk your elbows forward. (No momentum!)
- Place your feet up close to your bottom. It's necessary to have your legs apart on this one. (No momentum!)

These will help you get flexibility in your back. They are also good for beginners or those who have been doing straight-legged situps (which you should never do):
- Lie on your back with your knees bent and your feet on the floor; lift your chin to your chest time after time.
- Lie on your back with your knees bent and your feet on the floor; lift your head and shoulders without jerking and roll back down, time after time.
- Keep your arms out in front.

- Lie on your back with your knees bent and your feet on the floor; lift your head and your shoulders, and, with your arms at your sides, swing yourself off the ground from your waist so that you swing first one arm under your knees and then the other. Make it a smooth swing. Then roll smoothly down.
- Lie on your back with your knees bent and your feet on the floor; lift your head and shoulders and have your hands on your thighs. Now with a smooth motion, move first one hand toward one knee, and, as that hand comes down, slide the other hand up toward the other knee. Stay in position, swinging gently as long as possible, and then roll gently down.

To make the situp harder, make believe you have a very heavy trunk on either side of you. Put your arms out with hands placed against these very heavy trunks. Use all your strength to try to come up as you push these trunks along the floor. Be sure you breathe out with your mouth pursed as you struggle with the trunks. (See Figure 2.)

Figure 2

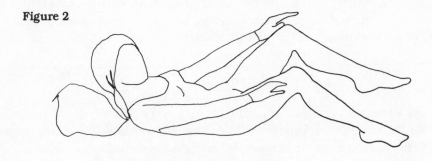

LEG LIFTS

Leg lifts are the most important exercises you can do for the most important supportive muscles of the belly wall. The lower part of the belly muscles take the most weight of pregnancies, of belly fat, and of sagging organs that cannot be contained in the bowl of the pelvis. Here are some excellent ways to exercise these muscles.

Practice situps for at least a couple of months or until you can do at least twenty-five situps in a row without strain, without your feet being held down, and without jerking yourself up off the floor, before you begin leg lifts. Leg lifts absolutely should *not* be performed or practiced if you have a painful lower back or if your back arches up off the floor as you try to lift or lower your legs. Any time you haven't been exercising for a while, go back at least several levels of exercise and work your way up again. Safety always pays off!

It is very important to keep the back of your waistline tight to the floor during the entire exercise. Every variation of the leg lifts done on the bed or floor requires that the back of the waistline be kept tight to the surface of the bed or floor.

The variations from the easiest leg lifts up to the hardest are as follows:

1. Lie on your bed with your knees bent, feet on the bed, chin on your chest. Bring one knee up to your chest, keep it there, and bring your other leg up. Raise both legs up over your belly and bring them toward your face alternately with a walking motion. (See Figures 3a, 3b, and 3c.)

Figure 3a

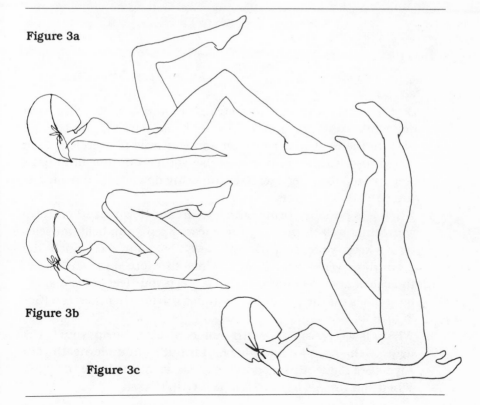

Figure 3b

Figure 3c

2. Lie on your bed with your knees bent onto your chest. Tuck your hands under the lower edge of your bottom. Lift your head and tuck your chin into your chest. Lift and straighten one leg and lower it to the bed, then lift that leg back to the chest and lower the other leg. (See Figure 4.)

Figure 4

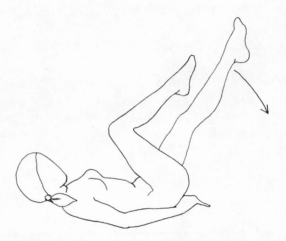

3. Do the same exercise with a straighter and straighter leg each day while continuing to keep your back down. If you tire, go back to the next easier version and continue to exercise. Each day start with the hardest exercise you can do but drop back step by step to easier exercises, tapering down till you really feel you can't do any more.

4. When it is possible, bring both legs up and down together. Keep your chin well down on your chest; keep your belly muscles tight; keep your back down! Never let your feet touch the ground or even come too close, since this forces the shifting of the pelvis and will arch your back. Keep your feet at least six to ten inches off the ground at all times during this exercise. (See Figure 5.)

5. When it is possible — with full control to keep your back against the floor — take your hands out from underneath your hips. (See Figure 6.) But **don't let your waistline leave the floor.** When you tire, go back to the next easier version.

6. When you're really getting good and strong, let your head down to the floor and continue to raise and lower your legs — back still tight to the floor! **Do not let your neck arch.**

   The minute you begin to feel as though you can't bring your legs up or let them down without arching your back up off the floor, go back step by step to easier versions. The more time you put in, even on the easier versions, the stronger your back and lower belly will become.

Figure 5

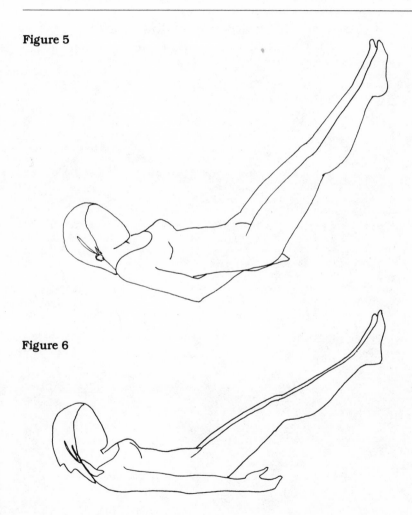

Figure 6

7. (For those who are very strong.) Head down, chin tucked into neck, arms out from under hips, raise and lower your legs. Keep them no less than six inches from the floor. See how long you can keep it up. Keep breathing steadily; don't hold your breath! Stop when you feel yourself weakening. Do not let your legs drop. Bring them to your chest or bend one leg to your chest while you bend the other to the floor. Back down tight to floor. Add weights to your ankles if you want to make it yet harder.

**Keep your back absolutely down tight
to the floor the whole time.**

⑨

The Upper Body

THE BREASTS

The consistency of the breasts changes constantly. They are affected by puberty, menstrual periods, weight gain and loss, sickness, general health, disease, childbearing, nursing, menopause, aging.

The breasts can get larger, smaller, firmer, softer. They can feel tender or painful; they can sag, unsag, develop large blue veins, leak colostrum, milk, and, in times of disease of the breasts, other fluids. During a period of nursing they can leak milk, they can ooze milk, they can stream milk, and they can spray milk.

The nipples can change from light to dark with puberty, with pregnancy, with nursing; they can change back to light with age. Hair often develops around the aureola (the outer ring of the nipple). The breasts can look like just nipples with no breast development, or they can be any size up to enormous and in some cases continue to grow — and grow and grow. They can be any shape, from conical to round, and point heavenward, point in opposite directions, point earthward (most common because of gravity); they can be shaped like pinnacles or pancakes or pendulums. Interestingly, *after* childbirth and nursing (at which time the breasts in some women get heavy and pendulous), in many cases the breasts pull back up and actually become restored in shape, though this may take several years. In aging, the breasts tend to pull back up. In a good weight-loss diet, the breasts sometimes pull back up; in a poor weight-loss diet, the skin sags and breasts most often only deflate.

A breast that is allowed to be pendulous and is given no support tends to have very poor circulation of blood and lymph; it is not unusual in such cases to find fungus infections in the fold between breast and chest.

In some women there is a tail to the breast that reaches well up under the arm. (See Figure 1.) As the years pass and the texture of the breast changes, this tail can make it appear that the muscles in this area are out of shape.

No amount of exercise is going to shape up the fatty glandular tissue of the breast.

No one has really symmetrical breasts — "a matching pair." Some women's discomfort comes from one breast being significantly larger than the other. The breasts still work just as well — and it does add a distinctive air to us. You are unique in a way that shows.

Figure 1

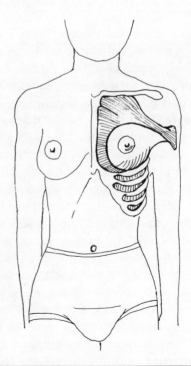

There are no magic formulas to even them up, but they can be made to appear evenly matched when you are dressed. This is by far the most sensible route for you to take. If you are embarrassed because uneven breasts call attention to you, pad the smaller side. Do you happen to be one of those people who get "hung up" on an idea and can't forget it? You could, if you feel you can afford to, try for breast enlargement on one side or breast tissue removal on the other side by plastic surgery.

Breasts of all shapes, sizes, and conditions can be benefited by the following piece of good advice:

Eat well, keep the muscles under the breast tissue in good shape, keep the breasts well supported, and then camouflage what you feel uncomfortable about.

CHOOSING A BRASSIERE

The Cooper ligament is all the support the breast has. This ligament is attached only to the skin of the breast and *not* to the chest wall at all! If the breasts are allowed to hang, gravity will slowly pull them down and they will lose shape and height and may stretch blood and lymph vessels, wrecking circulation and skin. Impact increases the pull of gravity. Unless you wear an excellent brassiere, the jarring impact caused by wearing high heels or running and jumping will break down breast tissue.

The blood supply that feeds the breasts comes in along the outside and the inside edges of the breast. If the blood supply is cut off, that part of the breast is essentially starved of food and will begin to show it by losing both solidity and tone. The flow of blood and lymph can be impaired both by the sag that comes about by not wearing a brassiere (if you have even a B-cup breast) or by wearing the wrong type of brassiere for you.

New students and faculty at the Massachusetts Institute of Technology have sometimes stared in amazement at the bulletin board ads for engineers for brassiere companies. But it *is* an engineering job to build brassieres, and it also takes some knowledge to choose the right brassiere for your particular breasts. You need to consider the purpose for which you are buying a particular brassiere; for example, if you increase in size at your menstrual period, you should certainly have a larger size to wear during that time. If you're going to be around the house, barefoot and relaxed, a soft bra with elastic straps is fine. If you have reasonably small breasts you still should have better than soft support when wearing heels, walking on hard pavement, or running.

If your breasts are cone-shaped, buy a brassiere that is cone-shaped. If your breasts are round, buy a rounded bra. Buy what suits your shape, not your taste. Do not distort the breast unnecessarily. Impaired circulation for whatever reason will finally take its toll. Try never to wear a brassiere that is too small for you either in depth of cup (or the breast will be squashed flat) or in circumference (or the entire breast will not be contained in the cup). Circulation is important in all parts of the breast.

The cup size must be considered separately from the band around the body. If the band is too loose, the entire bra will move up under your armpits in the back.

If your breast is not completely in the cup, the support will not be the best it could be. Be sure the underwire or any other part of the brassiere is not tight enough to cut off circulation at the points of blood supply. Women who are active should always try on brassieres till they think they've got the right one, then run in place and jump up and down to see if the breasts bounce. The less bounce, the less breakdown you can expect.

Women whose breasts are high up on the chest will usually have some difficulty finding a brassiere that is cut low enough under the arm for comfort. Keep searching. Try some that are made for wear with evening clothes. Try those made for running. Keep trying till you find what you need and feel comfortable in it. It is very difficult to encourage yourself to move freely when your brassiere cuts in across your underarm and upper back.

The heavier your breasts are, the more support you're going to need. Cotton cups are sturdy; shaped cups are sturdier; shaped, stiff cups are sturdiest yet. These are a godsend for very heavy-breasted women or women with painful breasts, since they afford some protection against bumps and hugs. If you are heavy-breasted or have painful breasts, you should wear a soft brassiere to bed for extra comfort. A sturdy cotton strap will help keep the cup from sagging and should, of course, be adjustable so that the cup can be lifted more as the material gives way. A strap-widener, which can be purchased from a notions store, will keep the brassiere strap from digging into the shoulder and causing pain. An underwire, which anchors a brassiere against your ribs, can be the greatest help of all against gravity. Don't give up if the first one hurts. Find one that doesn't. Pad it if you must.

If you are pregnant or have large breasts or wear heels or run, the right brassiere will

- prevent nerve damage or irritation;
- prevent breakdown of tissue;
- improve circulation;
- support the weight of the breasts;
- preserve symmetry;
- prevent injury from impact.

Choose a brassiere that has well-padded underwires for support, wide shoulder straps of nonstretch material, and stiff, molded, porous cups with a soft lining.

EXERCISE FOR SMALL BREASTS

If your breasts sag or are small, developing the pectoral muscles to make them shorter, thicker, and stronger will make the breasts seem larger and firmer.

To accomplish this, do the following:

Lie on your bed. Rest the upper arm on the bed and bend the elbow so that the hand is straight in the air. (See Figure 2.) Pick up your elbows and swing your arms in and down toward your thighs; circle them back up. Start making small circles, working slowly toward your thighs and back up; then circle in the other direction. Repeat this exercise in each direction a few times. Now, find the position where you feel the muscle is working most and work there.

Note: To trim down or to keep in shape, do just a few circles each day with light weights or no weights.

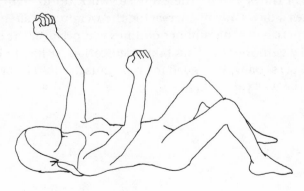

Figure 2

To increase the measurement of the chest, start with one-pound weights and work up over a period of time till you can do eight repetitions of the exercise before tiring. (See Figure 3.)

Figure 3

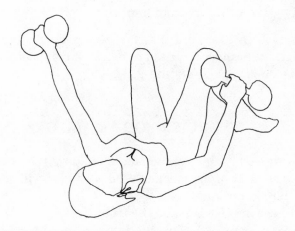

- Then, work up to eight repetitions each day.
- If you use adjustable plate weights, be sure to tighten the bolt with a wrench before each use.
- Keep a tight hold on any weights. If your hands get sweaty, dust them with powder.

If you are intent on gaining inches on your chest, increase the weights by a small amount every time you can, or increase the number of times you do the exercise. Work up to eight repetitions five times a day. Only by increasing the weights as often as you can and by increasing the number of times you perform the exercise will you really gain inches. This takes dedication. It has to be important to you personally. It is good for your muscles and local circulation and for the way you look.

KYPHOSIS, DOWAGER'S HUMP, AND ROUND SHOULDERS

Kyphosis, the forward curvature of the upper spine, can be caused by poor posture or loss of calcium. It can impair breathing and can cause neck, arm, and shoulder pain. It also restricts the lifting of the arms to the side or to the front. (See Figures 4 and 5.)

Dowager's hump is an unsightly, hormonally induced layer of fat that, in the middle years of some women, gathers right at the juncture of the neck and upper back. There is evidence that it may be genetic. It usually causes no physical problem.

Round shoulders are most often caused by poor posture. When you sit slumped or leaning forward working over a desk, the chest muscles contract, the upper back muscles stretch out, and the

Figure 4

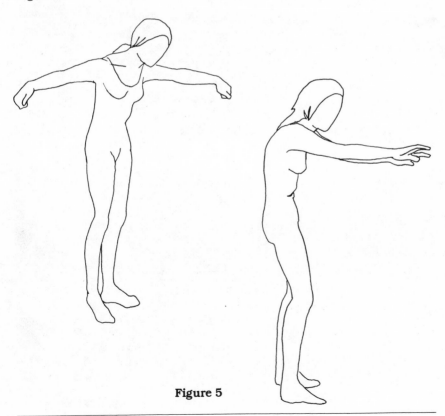

Figure 5

shoulders roll forward. The head and neck usually follow. This can cause impaired breathing and neck, arm, and shoulder pain. (See Figure 6.)

All of these conditions can be corrected to some extent. In the case of dowager's hump, the correction may be only visual, but sometimes the hump can be reduced slightly with weight loss. The sleeping position and the upper-body exercises from Chapter 14, The Twenty Most Important Exercises, will help produce a more upright upper back.

There is a point right between your shoulder blades that is hard to see, harder to reach, and almost always ignored. But it is very important! Just changing its position, as we will show you, can improve your breathing, improve the look of your chest, lift your breasts, increase your chest measurement by an inch or even two, straighten your shoulders, help relieve tense, painful neck, arm, and shoulders, slow down advancing kyphosis, and prevent dowa-

Figure 6

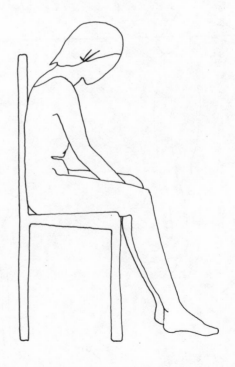

ger's hump from looking quite so obvious. It will also flatten your belly and take an inch to an inch and a half off your waistline. (See Figure 7.)

The shoulders themselves are not always involved in misshaping your upper body, but as you straighten that part of your back forward, your shoulders will hang more properly from their connections. They should not be forced back or hang forward, but should hang loosely.

If your shoulders have been round for a long time, you need the exercises from The Twenty Most Important Exercises to stretch chest-to-shoulder muscles and tighten back-to-shoulder muscles. Until the balance is made, the short chest muscles will try to pull your shoulders forward, like a short piece of elastic being stretched, and then, the minute you forget, *sproing!* Someone who has been round-shouldered for a long time can maintain an upright posture for only a short period of time. Are your shoulders like that?

Figure 7

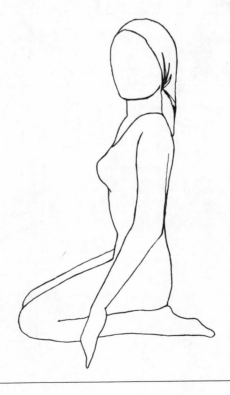

In addition to positioning at night and constant reminders to yourself during the day, use the upper-body exercises (when your back can be held straight). They will strengthen that part of your back. Afterward, that beautiful upper-back posture is easy — you no longer will be consciously aware of the fact that you are maintaining yourself upright.

If you have round shoulders, kyphosis, or a dowager's hump, you must stretch out the muscles across the front of the chest before you can reshape your shoulders, back, and chest to look the way you want them to and to work the way they should. This is necessary to maintain the flexibility of your shoulder joint while you straighten your upper back with other exercises and positions. Do this in bed — changing the body while you sleep is very effective and a really good use of time:

> Pin a folded face towel to the back of your pajamas where your back tends to bow out most strongly. If you're not allergic to tape, you can tape the towel in place. (See Figure 8.) While sleeping, remind yourself each time you roll over off your back to roll

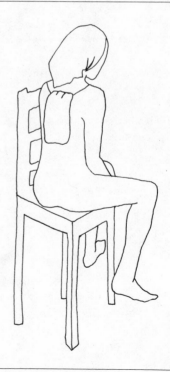

Figure 8

back onto the towel again. (It takes a while to institute these semiconscious commands.) Do not use a pillow under your head until your back is straightened up again. Sometimes that takes months! Pillows under your knees and lower legs will increase your comfort greatly and help to position your upper back.

This positioning gently eases and stretches out the shortened chest muscles that pull the shoulders in and down across the chest. Finally, you should be able to stand with your shoulders relaxed in the proper position. Some conscious effort goes into this position in the beginning till it becomes habit.

Exercise

In the morning grab hold of the headboard and pull down. This is a good exercise to use the important shoulder muscles while your back is still in the proper position from the flexibility gained from the sleeping position. Progress to the next upper-body exercises only when you can keep your upper back upright.

EXERCISE FOR BACKS OF UPPER ARMS

It is very difficult for most women to keep the muscles at the back of the upper arm firm. Many women always wear dresses with sleeves because they want to hide their flapping underarms.

With loss of weight, lymphedema of the arms, menopause, and aging, the problem will become worse unless you get into daily habits to prevent it from occurring. As with all body-related problems, prevention is better — and easier — than cure.

Here's a good exercise:

Sit in a sturdy chair with strong arms. Put your hands a little behind you on the arms of the chair and push yourself up with your arms and let yourself down again slowly. If this is tough for you, start by standing and, with your arms on the chair, let yourself down slowly. Put a pillow on the seat if you feel you might sit down hard, but don't do this variation at all if you think you're not strong enough to do it without falling. It's important to use only your arm muscles and not to let your thigh muscles help you. Put your feet farther out in front of your chair than you usually do to remind you to use your arm muscles.

When you feel quite strong and sure that you won't run into problems, stand with your back to a sturdy sink or table. Place your hands firmly on the edge. With your feet stretched out a little way in front, use the backs of your arms to support you while you lower your bottom into a sitting position and come back up again. The lower you let your bottom go, the harder the backs of your arms will have to work to raise you back up.

ELBOW INJURIES

The arms of women when hanging, elbows locked, thumbs out, makes a slight angle out over the hips. This is called the carrying angle but should *not* be used for carrying. (See Figure 9.) Be sure that you keep your elbows unlocked when you have weight on them or are going to hit a ball or carry anything. Straighten them as far as you can, then bend them very slightly. A locked elbow (elbow pushed completely back) is a dangerous position, one that leaves

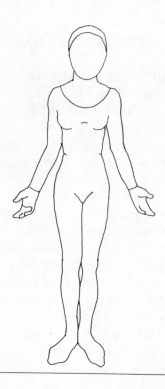

Figure 9

you open to injury. In this position you are using not muscle but ligament. Ligament if injured takes much longer to heal than muscle, since it has little blood supply. Muscle can take hard contractions and extensions. It is meant to do so. Be sure you use your muscles, not your ligaments, to bear mechanical stress.

LYMPHEDEMA OF THE ARMS

For many other reasons, but certainly after radical breast surgery, when the lymph system of the arm has been seriously disturbed, the lymph fluids may accumulate and cause the upper arm to swell in an uncomfortable and unsightly way. Lymph vessels will heal and auxiliary vessels will begin to work if you give them some encouragement.

The right positions can help the lymph fluids to drain. The right exercises can help force drainage and encourage development of new lymph vessels or recovery and reuse of the injured vessels.

The positions and exercises take little time or effort.

If you have lymphedema in the arms, sleep on your back with your arms up overhead resting on a pillow or pillows, being sure to keep your arms higher than your heart. (See Figure 10.) Or use

Figure 10

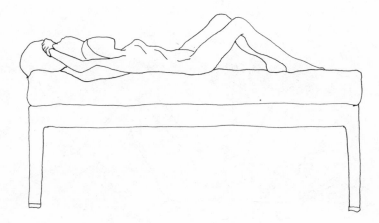

pillows on either side of you to keep your arms at your sides raised from the shoulder to the elbow. Put your hands across your belly. (See Figure 11.)

Figure 11

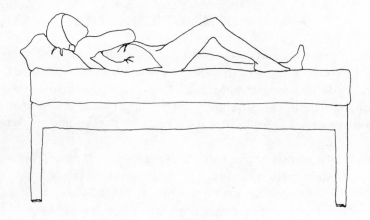

To institute faster drainage, raise your arms overhead and clench and unclench your hands over and over, or raise your arms, hands clenched, elbows bent up overhead, over and over. (See Figure 12.)

Figure 12

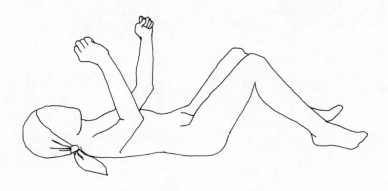

Do not do arm-swinging exercises. Centrifugal force will force blood and lymph fluids into the arm. Do not let your arms hang at your sides for long periods of time.

During the day rest the forearm often on top of your head while tightening and relaxing the muscles of your whole arm, time after time.

Do pushups against the wall, with your forearms (from the elbows to hands) high up the wall above shoulder level.

Push your hand or hands up against the roof of your car, or up against the top of the doorways, over and over. (See Figure 13.)

Make sure you wear a brassiere that does not cut into you, especially under your arm.

Do the towel-twisting exercise on page 186.

Figure 13

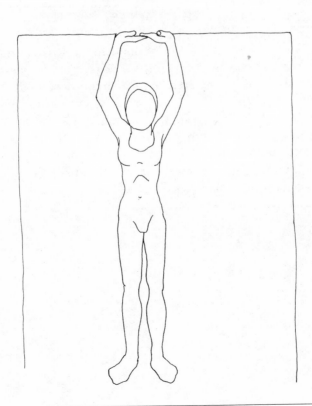

10
The Lower Body

HIP JOINTS

If you have a constant irritation in one hip joint, there may be one or several reasons. If you sleep on the side that aches, your problem may be caused by the joint pressing into a too-hard mattress. If it is the hip that is up that aches, you may have exceptionally wide hips or, again, a too-hard mattress, both of which force the knee that is reaching toward the bed to pull too hard, putting strain on the ligaments of the hip joint. The stretch is just too much, and a small irritation once begun becomes chronic because the cause of the irritation is left unchanged. (See Figure 1.)

Figure 1

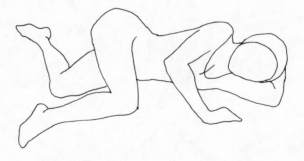

There are two ways to change things:

- For an aching hip against the bed, you need a soft mattress to relieve the pressure on the joint.
- For an aching hip on the upper side, either allow the other side of your hip to sink into the soft mattress or use a pillow between your knees to prevent your upper leg from *hanging* from the hip joint. Quite often just using the pillow between the knees makes the problem disappear. (See Figure 2.)

Watch the sort of seat you sit in. You'll often find that a certain kind of seat will make your hip ache. Get out of it! If the offending chair is in your home, find another to put in your favorite spot.

Keep track of just exactly what you are doing when you do hurt to find out what is causing the pain. Like a mystery story, follow leads and clues till you've tracked down the cause. For several days, keep a chart of when the painful periods with your hip begin. Once you have the earliest possible time that your discomfort starts (say, 12:00 noon) start a half-hour before that time to do this exercise, which will help undo the stress.

Exercise for Painful Hip

Place a thick phone book next to a strong bureau. Stand on it with the good leg; bend the knee slightly. Attach a small weight to your other ankle. (Lead weights from a hardware store may be wrapped in a cloth, which can be tied around your ankle.) Lean forward from the hips and swing your leg loosely forward and back, across in front and out to the side. Think of the leg as hanging *loosely like a pendulum* so that ligaments can gently stretch out. *If the weight you choose is too heavy*, the muscles will try to pull the leg back up

Figure 2

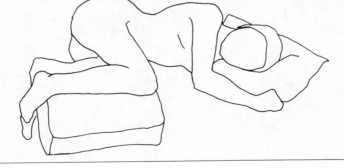

into the joint! To avoid this, keep the weight reasonably light — one to three pounds.

Obviously, you can't carry a phone book with you through your day's activities, but you still can do this exercise. Wherever you are, step up on the bottom step of some stairs, pretend there is a weight around your ankle, and swing your leg.

Running, jumping, and hopping are going to damage your hip until it is healed. Walk fast instead. Move around, but use both sides of your body evenly. Don't slump down into your hips while you are standing, and be sure not to lean into one hip.

EXERCISES FOR BACKS OF THIGHS AND BUTTOCKS

Unless you climb three or four flights of stairs a couple of times a day or jump rope often, the backs of your thighs — in fact, both entire thighs — are likely to be in poor condition. The following exercises will begin to get your thighs in better shape without great difficulty.

Lie on the floor with your feet about twenty inches up the wall or resting on a twenty-inch-high box. Start with your legs slightly bent at the hip and knee, and with your feet apart and turned in. (See Figure 3.) When you bend your knees, they should still move directly in a line over your feet and across your toes. Tighten just your bottom muscles first, till your bottom lifts itself off the floor. Tighten only till your waistline barely begins to lift. Relax your bottom to lower it to the floor.

Figure 3

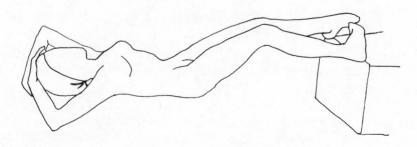

Variations

Before we begin the variations, you need to know that when your feet are pointed in, the inner sides of both thighs are exercised more; when the feet are turned out, the outer sides of the thighs are exercised more (see Figure 4); and when the feet are pointed straight ahead, the backs of the thighs will be well exercised. In each of the variations all parts of the thighs will be working a little, but some muscles will get more exercise, depending on the position of your legs. Feel the muscles with your hands to see if you're getting them tight where you want them tight. On all variations,

Try to use mostly your bottom muscles to lift your bottom off the floor. Keep your knees bent. Keep your waistline on the floor, and keep your elbows off the floor, arms and shoulders relaxed.

Figure 4

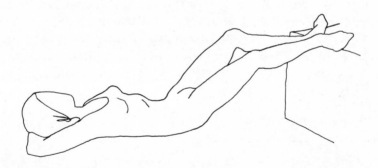

You should add tension to each of the variations as you can, by clenching the hip and thigh muscles hard. Continue to breathe steadily as you tighten the muscles harder. Try doing a few more variations each day with the feet turned in, out, and pointed straight ahead until you decide which ones you need most. Then do only them.

1. As you tighten your bottom to lift, and relax it to lower, pull your belly way in to separate the vertebrae more. Repeat four or five times. Change your foot position, first to straight ahead,

and repeat the exercise. Then turn the feet out and repeat the exercise. Continue to do this with each variation.

2. Blow out your breath with pursed mouth and use your tightened belly muscles to help lift.

3. Tighten both your belly and bottom muscles and lift.

4. Press on your pubic bone with your hands and lift.

5. Now, without hands on pubic bone, just make believe it's hard to lift. Harder! Keep breathing!

6. Place your feet side by side on the wall. Then try to tighten just one side of your bottom till it lifts up. Lower it. Then do the same with the other side. Move your feet farther down on the wall, still keeping them flat.

7. Try jumping both feet gently off the wall just a little way, and gently let your bottom come down to touch the floor each time.

8. Try gently jumping just one foot off the wall with the other leg bent up toward your chest. Do the same with the other leg.

9. Move in closer to the wall and repeat the whole routine.

10. Bend your knees while halfway in toward the wall with your bottom and repeat the routine again.

11. Now move your bottom all the way in toward the wall until it touches and repeat the whole routine in this position, first with your knees almost straight (you'll have to move your feet up the wall), then with your knees bent (move your feet down the wall).

12. To make each variation a little harder, use only the balls of your feet or just your toes on the wall except in the jumping variations.

Now that you've tried them all, choose the variations you need most and do them every day.

VARICOSE VEINS

Varicose veins can be caused by too little leg activity, weak connective tissue, or both. Because of the extra pressure they have to handle, the veins begin to expand and turn. Then they become longer and fold on themselves. Fortunately, this problem almost always starts where you can see it, and fortunately, there are things you can do to slow down and maybe even completely halt the process. The sooner you attack it, the better. Left alone, the condition will get more and more difficult to repair, with one problem always leading to another.

In the circulatory system, the blood that is pumped out of the heart returns to the heart. Blood travels away from the heart through the arteries to a network of smaller vessels called capillaries, from the capillaries into veins, and from veins back into the heart. The blood stays enclosed everywhere. Only in the capillaries do food and oxygen pass out of the blood to the body tissues and waste products pass into the blood from those tissues.

Arteries are thick-walled, muscular tubes that can stand much pressure. The thin-walled veins have little muscle in them; they are mainly elastic tubes. Thin flaplike valves along the veins, like doors that open only in one direction, let the blood flow toward the heart but stop it from flowing back.

Varicose means "unnaturally swollen or dilated," and that describes the condition of varicose veins. Actually, there are two sets of veins: one set just under the skin, and the other set between the muscles. The two sets are connected to each other by many short veins. Imagine the veins in your legs, one set under the skin, another set between the muscles, connected to each other in a one-way ladder arrangement: the blood can go only up in them if they're healthy; it can't go down.

Since veins aren't muscular, if you don't move you have only the pressure of the blood coming out of the capillaries to drive this column of blood up to the heart. If your job keeps you standing or sitting still for long periods of time, the veins fill up with blood. The valves, or little flap doors, will stop the blood from flowing back, but as you stand still or sit still, the pressure of the column of blood all the way up to the heart presses back down and blows up the veins with as much blood as they can hold.

The distance from your ankles up to your heart is about three and a half to four feet. That's a lot of pressure on those little elastic tubes. The veins between the muscles are supported by the muscles, so they don't blow up as much. But the veins under the skin are held much more loosely, so if you do a lot of quiet sitting or standing, sooner or later the walls of the surface veins will begin to spread. This spreading stretches the walls apart near the valves, creating pockets that fill with blood. The pressure pulls apart the valves even when they are "closed," and a little gap appears where the blood can flow back.

With the blood moving slowly in the veins, bacteria begin to gather in the little pockets at the sides of the valves, and inflammation sets in. The inflammation causes scarring. After a while, not only can the valves not prevent the blood from flowing backward, but even the forward flow is slowed up because of the scarring. As the flow slows, the veins become even more inflamed.

But let's see what happens when you exercise or move or even just shift your weight. The muscles of your legs tighten and relax, acting like a pump to squeeze the blood upward from the deep veins. While the muscles are relaxing, not only do the deep veins fill from the flow of blood from the capillaries, but the veins under the skin empty into the deep veins through the cross veins. This is the important part. Since the valves in the veins under the skin prevent the blood from flowing back down, the pressure drops in the part of the vein between the valves, as long as you keep pumping. This makes the pressure in the veins under the skin on your legs drop from three or four feet of pressure to anywhere from a few inches to about a foot of pressure, depending on how actively you move your legs.

Relieving Varicose Veins

The first sign of varicose veins is often a pain or ache behind the left knee. Tight panties, slacks, or girdles often result in an ache in the groin or in the legs, or both. Even if tight clothes don't make you ache, they cut off circulation to some degree.

To get relief, lie down. Elevate your hips on a folded towel and rest your legs on pillows that raise them higher than your heart. If your feet become numb or cold, or if you feel dizzy or faint, lower your feet by taking away a pillow or two.

While your legs are elevated, use your leg and foot muscles to pull the front of your feet up hard in the direction of your knees. Do this ten to twenty times.

If your legs are still aching, start massaging them gently from the foot toward the knee, still pulling the front of your foot up, time after time. Do both legs: even if only one aches, they're both in trouble. Always massage from the foot toward the knee.

The massage and pumping action of the feet, legs, and thighs helps to send the blood back up toward the heart; by elevating your legs, you allow gravity to help the process. For a change, you can push your feet alternately against a pillow, as if you're walking.

Try to rest several times a day with your legs and hips elevated. Work your feet till they stop aching, and then rest with them up for a while longer. Sleeping with your legs and hips elevated will be a great help.

When you are on your feet, it is important to wear loose clothing and flat, comfortable shoes. Anything that slows circulation or prevents free movement must be done away with; that means especially a girdle — unless your doctor has specifically recommended it for another problem — or panties or jeans or slacks that cut in at the groin.

Aching in Groin Area

Many women have aching in their groin area and never do catch on to what is causing it. Most panties have tight elastic across the groin. Girdles almost invariably cut in at the groin. Blue jeans and many other pants now made are much too stiff and too tight and cut into the groin when you squat or sit.

Clothing that cuts into the groin can seriously impair the return circulation from the legs. In turn, this can create local aching and can cause, or make worse, varicose veins.

Use clothing that is loose or clothing that stretches so easily that it never indents the skin.

This change of habit will positively benefit your health by improving your circulation whether or not tight clothes make you ache. If crotch-binding does not bother you now, it may later. Don't wait. Change.

Garters are, in effect, tourniquets. They severely cut drainage of blood back up from the feet and legs, which, because of gravity, already present a problem in drainage. Anything tight around the legs, especially in a band, will slow the flow of blood and cause the veins below the band to swell with the increased pressure. If you wear garters, or knee-high stockings with elastic tops, you have to move your muscles more rigorously to force the blood beyond that barrier. This back pressure also obviously puts a terrific strain on the walls of the veins.

Here are some important things to do if you have varicose veins:

- Remain as active as possible when you are on your feet by shifting your weight from foot to foot, coming up onto your toes and down frequently, coming up on onto your heels and down frequently.
- Rock when you are sitting or twist first one foot at the ankle and then the other, round and round. Keep your weight down to prevent too heavy a load on your circulatory system.
- Walk. Make it fun if you're able. Walk! Run! Jump! Dance!

Where your legs are concerned, either keep them moving or keep them up.

LYMPHEDEMA OF THE LEGS

As we saw in the last section, the supplying of oxygen and food for the cells and the taking-up of waste products happen at the capillary level. Where a capillary begins from a tiny artery, the blood pressure is higher than in the tissue through which the capillary goes, so some of the fluid from the blood filters out into the tissues. At the end of the capillary, just before it joins a tiny vein, the fluid pressure in the capillary becomes less than at the beginning, and as a result, the concentrated blood sucks fluid back in from the tissue by osmosis. But not all the fluid that seeped out from the capillary comes back in. A little is left over. And this little accumulates. So we have another branch of the circulatory system: the lymphatic vessels. These collect the excess fluid left over from the capillary filtering, and finally carry it back to the large veins. If the lymphatic vessels are blocked, then the tissue keeps swelling and swelling. That is called lymphedema.

If the lymphatics get partly blocked, the fluids begin to collect and you begin to notice some swelling, which is not only unsightly but uncomfortable. If all is going well, between two to five quarts of lymph move from the tissues back into the circulation daily. When all is not well in the circulation, feet and ankles can swell alarmingly and uncomfortably!

A lymph system that goes out of whack, due to surgery or disease, if forced constantly to practice the returning of fluid to the blood stream by exercise or general activity, seems, in the end, to develop extra vessels to help out.

There are many cases of complete recovery with no further problems. The most uncomplicated approach is to keep active or elevated the member that is troubling you. For lymphedema in any limb, be sure to elevate that limb for the night and as often during the day as it begins to swell. This uses gravity to help you drain it of fluid. (See page 13 for instructions on how to tilt up the foot of your bed for swollen feet, ankles, legs, or thighs.)

Put a pillow at the foot of the bed and walk your feet gently against it. (See Figure 5.) This helps to drain the feet and legs. If your feet are very delicate because of the swelling, try putting lamb's

Figure 5

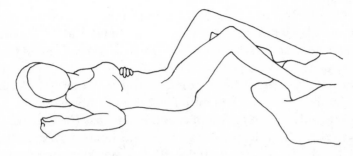

wool over the pillow. Exercises that keep the legs moving or elevated or both will help to relieve lymphedema if performed over a long period of time.

Caution: Do not do leg-*swinging* exercises. Centrifugal force tends to drive blood and other fluids to the legs and feet. Do not stand for long periods (especially without moving), because this tends to make the blood and other fluids pool in the feet, under the force of gravity.

Try to keep fluids from collecting in your feet and ankles. Your body parts can get into bad habits, too. The only way to break a bad habit is consistently to prevent it from expressing itself. Try to prevent swelling by shifting constantly from foot to foot. As soon as you see or feel any swelling, lift the affected part so that it can drain. At the same time, start a pumping action, by pushing rhythmically against something, to help the drainage. Use a wall, pillow, floorboards, or floor.

Caution: Limbs in which you have lymphedema must *absolutely not* be massaged. The tissue is already swollen and delicate. Massaging will only serve to break down more tissue. Use only drainage and exercise until the limb has behaved normally for several weeks.

"CELLULITE" AND "SADDLEBAGS"

Many people confuse "cellulite" and "saddlebags." Saddlebags refer strictly to the loose muscles that hang off the buttocks and thighs for lack of the proper exercise. This condition gives you a very large, loose behind and a large measurement around the upper part of your thighs. Saddlebags are reasonably easy to get rid of through exercise.

Cellulite is the filling of the fat cells that overlie our thigh, buttock, and belly muscles. This formation of fat and fluid in just these areas is common to many women because of a hormonal fatty apron called paniculus adiposus. These fat cells are like many flattened balloons until, with misuse, disuse, and poor diet, we fill them with fat and fluids. Cellulite is difficult, but not impossible, to get rid of.

The only way to get rid of cellulite is to lose the excess fluids and fats in those fat cells through a combination of a very strict diet and very hard exercise. Admittedly, it's a long, slow process, but it is certainly worth the effort.

Your diet must be low in calories and in refined sugars and starches to help you lose the stored fat. It must be low in salt and high in potassium to help you lose the stored fluids. Bowels must be kept open and regular, and no laxatives should be used except in emergencies. Most laxatives deplete the body of potassium; the lack of potassium causes fluids to be retained. If you have to take a diuretic ("water pill") under doctor's orders, be sure to compensate by increasing still more your intake of foods high in potassium. You need the potassium to help you lose fluids naturally. Instead of using laxatives, promote regularity by eating foods high in roughage, or try the recipe for seed cereal in Chapter 17.

Along with the diet, you must start exercising to improve the circulation in your lower body. Increase the movements gradually; then increase not only the number of movements but the force you put into them. Look at the legs of women who are heavily into swimming, mountain climbing, bike riding, or tap dancing. This much work should not be necessary once you have accomplished the eradication of the cellulite, but these activities do help you to rid yourself of this unsightly problem much faster.

KNEES

A woman has a greater angle of the femur, or large thighbone, because her pelvis is wider than a man's. This angle causes no problems for most of us, but if you have knee troubles, particularly if you are overweight, this angle means that additional stress is put on the knee joint. When the inside ligaments of the knee are stretched, in time all the soft tissues of the knee joint, and even the bone, will change shape from the additional stress. Eventually, this can cause you to become extremely knock-kneed. (See Figure 6.) This stress at an angle can also result in hip and foot problems. Placing your feet directly under your hips by keeping the feet a little apart will remove a lot of the stress on the knees and the foot arches. (See Figure 7.) This position is easier on the knees and the feet in any case, even if you are not overweight. It also provides you with a position that is better for balance and an easier one from which to move to a new position.

Figure 6

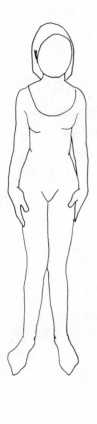

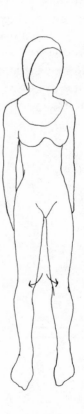

Figure 7

Crossed legs increase the stretching of the ligaments of the in-side of the knee. (See Figure 8.) Instead, when you sit, try to put your legs up on another chair, a coffee table, an ottoman, or desk drawer — anything available of the right height, which is about knee-high.

In women, knock-knees are most often caused by overweight. During the teen years especially, when the bone ends are going through a rapid growth period, excess weight can distort the knees for a lifetime. As we have seen, the wideness of the hips makes any extra load on the thighbones produce an inward-directed push at the knees. This is compounded because, as young girls, we are taught to keep our thighs together. Athletics can offset the problem, sometimes completely, but exercising when you are significantly overweight can create its own problems. The very best you can do for yourself (or for your daughters) is to keep the body during the teen-age years as free of extra fat as you can. Problems with knock-knees can occur later in life, but it usually takes considerably greater weight gain to distort the bone ends once they are fully developed.

It seems obvious that, in order to walk and squat with your feet under your hips, to sit without crossing your legs, to move in any direction comfortably and easily, slacks are the answer.

Figure 8

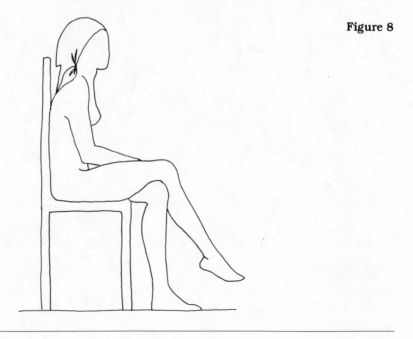

BOW LEGS

Poor standing posture, wearing high heels, and, in some women, either looseness of knee ligaments or lack of strength in muscles surrounding knees may cause a bow-legged effect.

Of course there are "true" bow legs, but more often than not the appearance of bow legs can be quickly corrected with a change in posture. Tuck under your bottom, turn your feet out slightly, and unlock or bend your knees very slightly. If you've become used to standing with overstretched ligaments, this new posture will feel strange. Get used to it! In almost every case the new position will not only benefit your appearance, but will in the long run prevent your having knee problems, large upper thighs, and, in time, an aching back.

There are two surfaces, or runners, on which the knee joint moves. When you let the knees lock all the way back, the outside runner is already locked in place and the inside edge continues forcing its way back till it, too, is locked back. The extralong runner forces a twist in the leg, which leaves you with a bow-legged appearance. Try standing in front of a mirror and watch how, as you lock your knee back, it causes the leg to twist in and the knee to twist toward the center and then back. The twist will be much more visible in some because the ligaments have already been stretched. Keeping your feet turned slightly out, your bottom tight, and your knees always unlocked will help with your posture in general, not just with bow legs.

MUSCLE SPASMS OR CRAMPS IN CALVES

Muscle spasms most commonly occur in the calf, in the middle of the night. They can be caused by a number of things: exercising more than usual or not exercising enough. They can also be the result of a general circulatory problem or a poor diet. If you have had them, you know they are no laughing matter; they can be wicked. The walls of larger and smaller veins that communicate between skin and muscle, possibly already weakened, can actually burst when the flow of blood through them is blocked by the muscle cramp. If you have varicose veins or spider veins, you must be careful about how you work out the cramp. Forceful kneading may cause bleeding or make worse any bleeding that may have occurred.

Getting Out of Bed with a Leg Cramp

Keep a bath towel by the side of your bed. If you get a cramp, put the towel around the ball of the foot that has the cramp and pull on it gently until you can force your knee to straighten out. (See Figure 9.) Then, as the cramp loosens, elevate your feet with a pillow and massage gently through the cramped muscle toward your heart. (See Figure 10.)

Figure 9

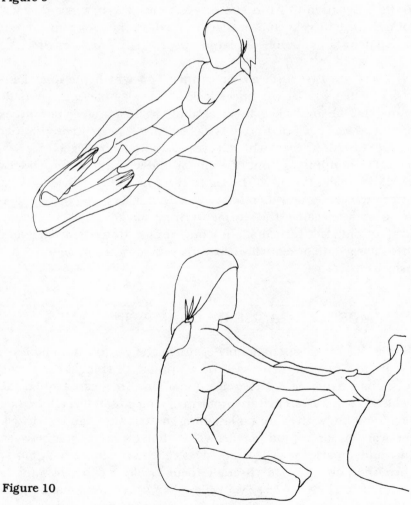

Figure 10

Next, take your feet off the pillow and walk them gently against the pillow for about five minutes. (See Figure 11.) Stop every half-minute or minute and pull the towel around the bottom of the foot of the cramped leg and pull up gently, as before.

Figure 11

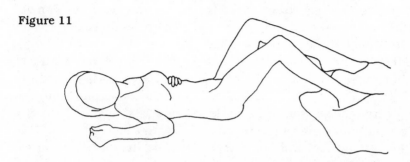

A really severe cramp can pull your heel up so hard that it's difficult to get your heel down onto the floor to stretch the cramp out. If that happens, take hold of the front of your foot with your hand. Pull your toe up and stretch your heel down. (See Figure 12.) Since your leg muscles and the spasms or cramps in them will be very tight, you probably won't be able to undo them completely or move your toe and heel very far.

As soon as you can pull the toe up even slightly, get your whole foot flat on the floor. This will feel awful for a few minutes, but it's the best way to get the cramp undone.

Figure 12

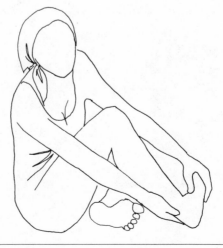

Take a step with the uncramped leg forward, knee bent, with your hands leaning in toward the wall or on a barre. Keep your head up and bounce the heel of the cramped leg *gently* down toward the floor little by little till you can get the heel down to touch the floor. (See Figure 13.) Move the uncramped leg farther forward. The farther back you can get the cramped leg, the more stretch you can get and the better you can undo the cramp. The position calls for head up, chest up, bottom in, heel stretching down.

After the muscle is stretched out, lie down and elevate both feet and knead the muscle where the cramped area was, massaging gently through it toward the heart so that the blood flow that was cut off through the cramped muscle can now be eased, with gravity and massage, back through the muscle toward the heart.

Now get up and walk around for at least five to ten minutes. Don't just stand! Walk! Don't run, hop, or jump; that may make your leg cramp up again. Every once in a while stop and stretch the cramped leg back as far as possible, leaning your hands against a wall, as before.

Figure 13

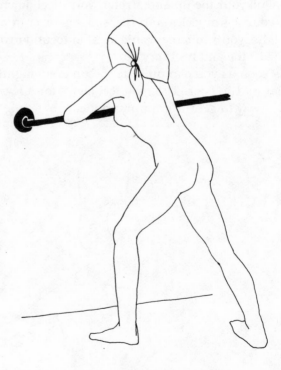

Other Aids for Muscle Spasms

It also helps if you can climb into a warm tub for a while, or use a heating pad behind the knee. If you want to try to stop leg cramps from occurring, there's a good chance that improving your circulatory system in general will also help relieve this condition. A walk before bedtime is a good idea. If you can't walk on your feet, walk against the pillows in bed. If you get cramps often, *make the walking a habit!*

Yes, overexercising can also cause leg cramps, so *don't overdo.* Work your way up gradually — just one minute or so more every day of exercises that keep your legs moving. Force yourself gradually to get out of the habit of standing or sitting still for long periods. If you must sit, use a rocking chair. If you must stand and wait, walk around — or just shift your feet often while you are standing. In bed, walk your feet against pillows. Lying down with legs elevated several times a day for just five minutes will also help.

Start with each of these suggestions very slowly and gradually and work up. For only the first few days or a week when you begin to exercise, you may have a few more leg cramps than usual. Then, as your body readjusts, you should have fewer and fewer.

BUNIONS OR HALLUX VALGUS

When the capsule between the muscles and the joint of the large toe where it connects to your foot becomes irritated and swollen, you are said to have a bunion. It is, simply, bursitis of the large toe joint, and is quite often very painful. It is usually associated with a deviation of the big toe toward the other toes, a condition called hallux valgus, which is a serious deformity of the joint of the large toe. Generally, the term bunion is applied not only to the painful bursitis but also to the deformity. (See Figure 14.)

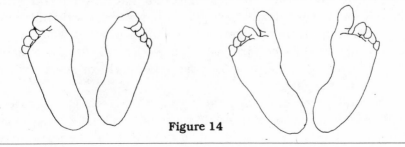

Figure 14

What Causes a Bunion?

Any kind of footwear that pushes the large toe in toward the other toes and out of line with the large toe joint is bound to start an irritation. This can start an overgrowth of bone, leading to a seriously deformed and painful foot.

Shoes with narrow or pointed toes, short shoes, high heels, shoes that are too narrow, ballet shoes that are too short or too narrow, all can cause problems, as can stretch stockings or socks or nonstretch stockings or socks that are simply too small.

Can Bunions Be Prevented or Corrected?

Obviously bunions can be prevented. Correcting a bunion is simple but does take time. It is not necessary in many cases for the large toe joint to remain grossly deformed or irritated.

What Do You Do First?

Put away all those shoes and socks and stockings that are causing your problem. Buy yourself some slightly longer, broad-toed, flat, soft shoes, a box of rolled absorbent cotton, and some adhesive tape. Put enough cotton between the large toe and the second toe to ease them slightly apart without causing any discomfort. If the big toe still presses the cotton and the other toes, place a piece of tape around the foot, just below the bunion, firmly enough to help the toes spread. Wear the cotton between the toes day and night. Add a slightly larger wad of cotton each time you can with comfort. When the large toe is finally adjusted to being straight out from the large toe joint, keep that size wad between the toes for several weeks. If you have had an overgrowth of bone and the joint looks large and is tender, it may take several weeks for the soft tissue to fill in on the inside of the joint. When it does fill in, you may find that you need a slightly longer shoe. It will help to ensure proper growth and stability of the joint if you continue to keep the cotton between the toes when you sleep or when you wear shoes in which it will not show.

Try not to go back to styles of shoes or socks or stockings that will irritate the joint.

If you feel you must wear the wrong shoes for a party, travel to and from the party in comfortable shoes that will not injure you and carry the "bunion makers" in a bag to be put on when you arrive.

Then sit as much as possible. Want to dance? Why not barefoot?

Now comes the important part. To develop or to redevelop the right muscles to hold the toe in its proper position, you must do the following exercise often. Only when the muscle has been strengthened will the toe remain in its new position without the help of the cotton. With the cotton taped where it belongs, start running gently in place, pushing down as hard as you can with your big toe and the one next to it. Do not use the other toes. If you do not want to run, use one hand to steady yourself on a table or sink and just come up as high as you can on your big toe and the toe next to it and down. Repeat as many times as you can, being sure to press both toes hard into the floor each time you come up on them.

PAINFUL METATARSALS

Putting your foot into a shoe with a heel of any height that elevates your own heel places the weight of your body on the heads of the metatarsals (the bones that run back from the toes to the instep). This position tilts open the joints between the metatarsals and the toes, and lets your weight bear down on the opened edge of the heads of the metatarsals. The higher the heel, the more of your weight rests on those bones and the less you are capable of using the muscle to hold that part of your foot in the proper position. For instance, if you stand on your toes, you can't last too long without resting your heels back down on the floor again. A high heel keeps the heel of the foot raised while allowing the muscles to relax. This stretches ligaments in your feet that weren't meant to be stretched. If your metatarsal bones have been forced down (you can usually see by the calluses on the soles of your feet), try wearing rubber thong sandals so that the metatarsals can build small hollows for themselves. This shape allows the muscles and ligaments around the metatarsals to adjust while you walk, The gripping of your toes tends to tighten the muscles and pull the metatarsal bones back into position.

A bare foot is most natural and best. If a foot is always allowed its freedom and you walk on sand, grass, or wood, your foot usually preserves itself in a healthy condition. A lot of barefoot-type action is really necessary to keep the feet healthy. A flat sandal with a

Figure 15

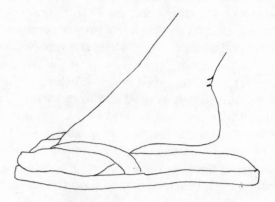

rubber sole and plenty of room for the toes to move is next best, if only to protect the foot from hard pavements and dangerous litter. (See Figure 15.)

11

The Face and Neck

FACE EXERCISES

Your mouth has a wide band of muscle in a ring around it and then muscles (eleven pairs!) attached to it at different points to keep it in place and to help it to do its job. (See Figure 1.) If these muscles get weak and begin to sag, the skin covering them will sag too.

Figure 1

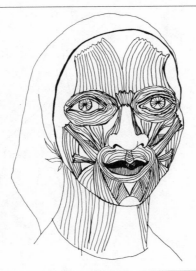

Like the other sphincters of your body, your mouth is meant to tighten and relax like the opening of a purse or sack. But in addition to controlling the mouth's opening and closing, the muscular attachments enable it to move around so that you can clear food from different portions of your mouth and stabilize your food to some extent while you chew. Most important, the muscles enable you to speak and to touch. These movements alone do much to keep your facial muscles healthy.

Here's an exercise that will improve the tone of these muscles even more. Place your thumb inside your cheek to feel the ring of muscle. Move your thumb farther into your mouth till it is under the so-called laugh line that develops from nose to mouth. Now, with great contractions, slowly tighten or purse your mouth as hard as you can over your thumb. (See Figure 2.) Relax slowly and tighten it again. It's rather strange and interesting to find that the muscles of your face can also get stiff.

Move your thumb around slowly from place to place along the edges of this sphincter muscle and tighten your mouth slowly and hard over your thumb in each position. The muscles attached to the top of the sphincter pull upward close to the nose, a little catty-cornered out toward the upper outside of the muscle, out to the

Figure 2

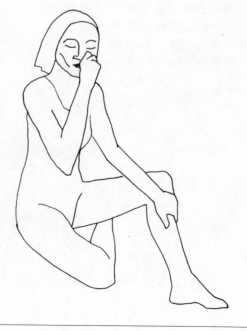

sides from the side of the mouth muscle, and downward from the bottom of it. When you're doing this exercise, your mouth should always pull in and against the thumb and teeth — hard! Relax it slowly and repeat. It is the repetition of the exercise that does the job of preventing loose muscles.

Tightening any muscle slowly and as hard as possible tends to make it a little thicker. This will help to fill out the skin again, but you've got to do it a lot.

The muscles around your mouth will often begin to sag seriously if you have had your teeth removed. Artificial teeth at best can do only about a quarter of the work that your real teeth can do.

Here's an exercise that is good for anyone, but especially for people who wear dentures. All you have to do is practice chewing on an infant's teething ring. Chew gently to begin with, then a little harder each day, moving the ring all the way around your mouth so that each section of your teeth gets to chew on the ring. (See Figure 3.) Build up daily till you can apply a lot of pressure and feel your teeth clamping hard and your jaws clenching as hard as possible, even if you wear dentures.

Figure 3

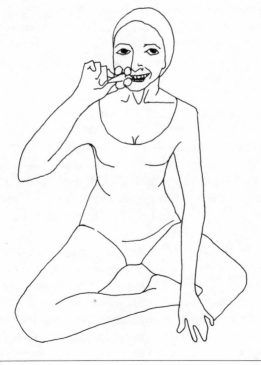

Now start using your teeth on natural substances that are chewy, such as meats, raw vegetables, and so on. Chew them into a fine mush. More chewing also adds more enzymes from the saliva, which helps keep your teeth cleaner. This is good practice whether you have natural teeth or dentures.

DRY SKIN AND WRINKLES

Lack of muscle tone is not the only cause of sagging facial skin. Your face also may begin to sag when you have lost a lot of weight very suddenly. Sometimes this is from a diet too low in protein and sometimes it is merely the skin sagging when a lot of fatty tissue has been lost from between the facial muscles and the skin, as in menopause or with the use of a weight-loss diet.

Drying makeups can dry the skin enough to cause lines without breakdown of muscle. Dry houses and climates can pull moisture out of your skin. A humid atmosphere keeps your skin moist and helps prevent wrinkling.

If the climate you live in is dry, if you have central heating, if your skin tends to be dry, get yourself a humidifier, but not one of the little vaporizers that give you a quart or two of water. An effective humidifier should hold from eight to twelve gallons and should take care of one room for a half-day per filling during a cold winter. If you are trying to keep your skin in the best of condition, you should have a big humidifier in each room where you spend time. Look for quiet ones. If you've got to live with it, you don't want to be constantly aware of it. Humidifiers must be kept very clean. Bacteria and molds grow on moist surfaces; unless they are cleaned off weekly, they will multiply in the damp air and make the room smell.

Washing the humidifier once a week with a dilute solution of a strong bleach and then rinsing well works, or you can use the commercially available bacteriacides. The humidifier is a most important adjunct to healthy skin.

Your skin is affected by the soaps you use. Detergents do much damage to many people's skin. Make sure you use only real soaps, not just for washing yourself but also your laundry. Lying on detergent-washed sheets for six to eight hours every night can have a very bad effect. Drying yourself on detergent-washed towels can damage your skin. You have a natural protective oily covering on your skin that can be easily broken down by penetrating detergents.

Be sure to wash your face with lots of water to keep your face moist. While it is still wet, cover your face with a fine layer of oil (without preservatives) to keep the moisture in. Oil helps to keep your face from wrinkling by preventing moisture from escaping.

It is not necessary to use soap on your face more than once a day unless your job is a very dirty one. Never use a detergent bar to clean your face. The natural protective balance that your face goes to so much trouble to produce should not be destroyed. Detergents — all of them, to my knowledge — will destroy this protective layer. Using a simple bar of pure soap (the one that floats is pretty good) is the most extreme washing treatment you should give your face. A soft, natural toothbrush is much less expensive and gets into smaller crevices than a complexion brush. Rinse the toothbrush and leave it out where the light can get to it between washings. (Light and air kill bacteria.) If your facial skin is very fragile or seems to be in a separated layer from the muscle underneath, the tooth-brush is out for you.

Do you try to hold your face still to prevent wrinkles? That's no way to live. Don't try to sleep with your face out of your pillow; just make sure that you wash your sheets in soap rather than detergents. Add more oil to your face before bed if you want. Get small-patterned, multicolored pillow slips so that the oil won't show. Lean your chin on your hand when you sleep, if you want. If you're eating enough protein and chewing hard and talking, laughing, and singing, your face is going to remain in better condition longer.

Sleeping or resting with your feet a little higher than your face will allow gravity to tip more blood into the face and scalp. Use a slant board (if you want to spend the money) or just tilt up the foot of your bed. If the tilt disturbs you for any reason, put pillows under your feet, knees, and hips to elevate them instead.

If you walk briskly or run in place for a while before lying down with your feet up, you will speed the flow of blood to the face and scalp.

EXERCISES FOR AND CARE OF NECK

If you look at the necks of older women, you can see that in general the skin of the neck begins getting "crepey" before the facial skin has shown many changes. Notice where the neck turns — over the edge of a turtleneck, on both sides of a choker — when the chin is dropped.

Your neck has very few oil glands. If you don't live in a grimy city, you should wash your neck with soap no more than once a week. Some kind of good oil — vegetable oil or an oil-based form of Vitamin E — should be applied to a wet neck in the evening and if possible in the morning. Jutting the chin forward to tighten the muscles for this activity is an effective exercise for loose skin on the neck.

Diet is always most important. High-protein, low-fat diets are sometimes too low in fats. This will cause skin to dry and wrinkle. Remember: good skin comes from both the inside and the outside.

If you hate your loose neck skin, try not to wear clothes or jewelry that pull against the skin of your neck or clothes around your neck that absorb the oil you need so badly in that area. Increase circulation to the neck by sleeping and resting with the foot of your bed tilted up. This is an even more advantageous position right after you've slowed down a little after strenuous exercise, because circulation is already increased.

Never let your head arch back. If you lean your head back when the vertebral arteries are at all constricted as they go up the back of the neck and into the skull, you may constrict them further, making you dizzy or nauseated, or even causing yourself to pass out.

If you have suffered a neck injury, are very out of shape, or get dizzy easily, do these *only* with your doctor's OK. Stop if you begin to feel dizzy! If you can, do all these exercises sitting cross-legged on the floor with your back straight, hands on your ankles, and shoulders down and relaxed.

1. Always do this exercise *first and last.* Drop your head onto your chest, relax, sigh a big sigh. Let your head roll loosely, *completely relaxed,* from shoulder to shoulder. *Beginners* should do only this one exercise for a few days or weeks.
2. These are stretching, relaxing, and building exercises. Do these variations five to ten times each and every day.
   a. Turn your head from side to side, with your nose over your shoulder. (See Figure 4.)
   b. Bend your head from side to side, leaning your ear toward your shoulder. (See Figure 5.)
   c. Bend your head forward onto your chest and back up. (See Figure 6.)

Figure 4

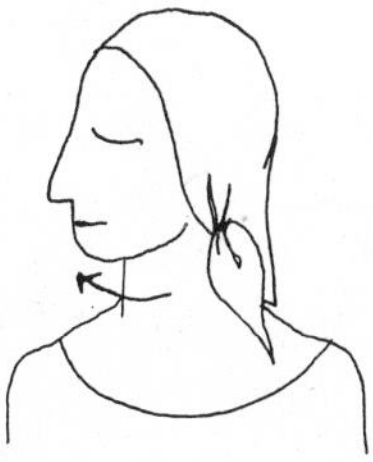

Figure 5

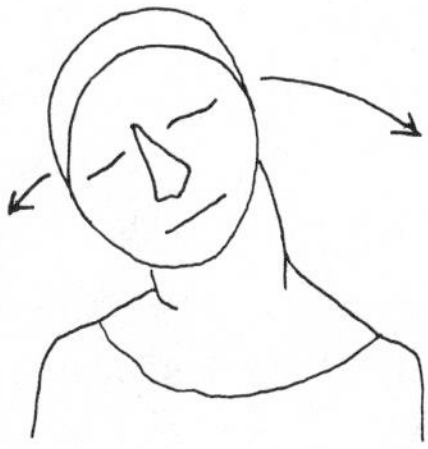

Figure 6

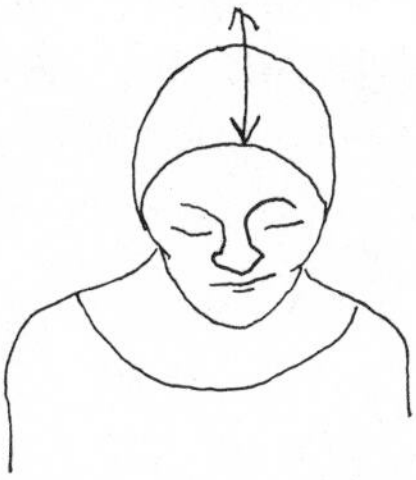

Figure 7

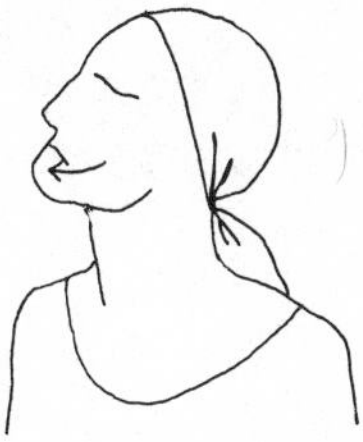

d. Repeat all of the above (a through c) with gentle opposing pressure from one hand against the direction in which the head is bending.
3. The next two are for double chins.
  a. Turn your head to one side, then stretch your neck along your shoulder. Jut your chin far forward. (See Figure 7.) Making chewing movements, jut your chin forward each time you chew.
  b. In the same position, open your mouth wide. Jut your chin way up and close your mouth. Keep chewing this way.
4. Repeat each of the following exercises five to ten times a day.
  a. Pull both your shoulders up into a shrug, then down level, and then far down.
  b. Roll one shoulder loosely around forward in a circle and then back. Then roll the other shoulder loosely around in a circle and back.
  c. Roll both shoulders loosely around in a circle forward and then back.
  d. Turn one arm and shoulder forward while turning the other back. Alternate looking each time toward the palm that is turned up.
5. Once again, let your head drop onto your chest. Relax, sigh a big sigh, and roll your head loosely from shoulder to shoulder.

LIVER SPOTS

Many of us develop brown spots, "liver" spots, on our hands and face especially. These spots look like light freckles, small or large, and tend to appear after we've passed the age of thirty. They will sometimes appear, as will also a brown-mask effect on the face, if you use the Pill and sometimes, but much less often, when you're pregnant. In many cases, you can make most of them disappear totally by spreading the contents of Vitamin E capsules over them daily for a few months; they will gradually lighten until they vanish. Spreading Vitamin E over the face and hands daily is a good habit in any case, because it also helps to keep the skin moist. Some Vitamin E should be taken internally also.

12

Exercises
for Heart and Lungs

WALKING

Walking is a *natural exercise,* the single best exercise for most people. It uses many muscles and can be managed by almost everyone.

Walking speeds up your heartbeat comfortably; you breathe faster and the blood courses through your body; your muscles stretch and contract; your bones twist and turn in their joints and sockets. Every body process is speeded up in a comfortable and natural way. A good *daily* walk will almost always lower both your average blood pressure and your average pulse rate after several weeks. If you walk fast for a half-hour every day, you can lose about twenty-four pounds a year without changing your diet.

There is good reason for the old phrase "Walk it off." Walking reduces tensions almost miraculously. Try to build up to walking at least an hour a day. *Never* walk when you have a fever or a headache, but try not to postpone walking for more than a day unless you're sick. If you have a circulatory disorder and are worried about cold being a vasoconstrictor, remember that walking is a vasodilator. Just dress more warmly than you usually do and put a scarf around your face to breathe through. If you're going to go for a walk outside and, for any reason, you doubt your ability to return safely, take a friend with you. Better yet, stay in and walk in place behind your chair. If you have any signs of sickness, stop. Start again when you're better.

Walk outside if you can. Do you remember how it feels to walk barefoot on the grass? Try it! The ground is bumpy and uneven, and the grass is a natural cushion. A soft, pliable, uneven surface will get you used to the unexpected. Go barefoot as much as you can; your feet, if they're normal feet, work better if you do go barefoot. If you can't go barefoot, wear flexible shoes with air holes in the uppers. If you begin to get blisters, cover and protect them immediately to prevent them from getting worse. Vitamin E from an opened capsule applied to blisters that have broken stops the burning sensation.

Bare feet, of course, can't "run down at the heels." Your toes are used more when you are barefoot and your foot can roll forward freely and naturally. Your feet not only support your body and carry you about, but the arches act as a built-in set of shock absorbers.

The less noise your feet make as they come in contact with the ground, the less you will jar your spine. Thick soft soles absorb impact, as do bent knees and grass. Between each separate bone of your spine, each vertebra, is a disc, an area with thick gelatin-like liquid, surrounded by tough fibrous cartilage. These discs act as shock absorbers or cushions. With age or with misuse, the discs often get thinner, shock absorption lessens, and the wearing on the bony parts can cause pain. Think of the discs as balloons, and walk in such a way as to prevent heavy shocks to these balloons. A floating or soft springy action, rather than a jarring action, is what you should ease into. Bouncing will be fine once you learn to use your arches, knees, hips, and spine. You have seen slow-motion pictures of a good gymnast on a trampoline. Start with conquering the "floating" action; your body then will automatically know how to bounce lightly.

Really stretch out. Walk fast and hard for a few minutes; you'll soon hit a natural stride and pace. Trying a bit harder than usual is a good way to gauge just how much you can do. Your body will fall naturally into what is comfortable for it. In fact, you can tell what your natural gait is by sitting on a table and dangling one leg straight down over the edge, letting it swing passively. The number of swings it makes per minute is the same as the number of strides it takes per minute if you walk without any strain.

Try to relax consciously while walking. Sounds funny? Once it has become a natural thing for you to walk, it is natural to relax while you walk. Until then, think about it and do it purposely.

Wear comfortable clothes — clothes that stretch and absorb but that can be opened up or removed if you get too warm. In cool weather, wear a hat and gloves to increase retention of body heat. Most people who walk a lot carry at least a little something with them in case they — or the local dogs they may bump into — get hungry. Take fruit for yourself and a pocketful of dog biscuits for the animals.

Listen to your body. You must be the final judge of how you feel. Soon after you have walked you should feel not tired, but elated. After you have been at it a while, you will be able to sense very small differences in your body. To a very large degreee, the people around us learn how to live from our example. So walk with them. You'll be building habits that will improve your life, their lives, and the lives of their husbands, wives, children, and friends. A real legacy almost anyone can give.

Here are some tips on how to get the most out of walking, no matter where, or for how long, you do it.

1. Wear flat shoes. They will automatically improve your balance and posture.
2. Keep your feet always in line with your hips and your knees. Bend your knees and check to be sure you can look down and see your big toe on the inner side of your knee.
3. Keep your pelvis tucked under, your bottom tight.
4. Bend or unlock your knees very slightly. This will help you use your thigh muscles and keep your pelvis tucked under.
5. Tighten your bottom hard with each step — the right buttock when the right foot goes down; the left when the left foot goes down.
6. Tighten your lower belly.
7. Lift your chest.
8. Inhale a little more than you usually do; exhale a little more than you usually do.
9. Keep your head up and your chin slightly in.
10. Keep your shoulders down and loose and let them swing for balance.

JOGGING, THE PROS AND CONS

Women are lucky. We do not have the life-or-death need for cardio-pulmonary work that men have. Our systems seem to be much more elastic. With a full uterus and up to sixty-five extra pounds we seem to be able, in the majority of cases, to breathe perfectly adequately and to circulate even more blood than we do when we aren't pregnant, and in a very efficient manner. Men's cardiovascular systems do not have this elasticity. With stress and lack of physical activity, men start to become incapacitated, even to die, in their twenties and thirties, most often from cardiovascular problems.

Although serious cardiovascular problems generally do not occur in women until after menopause, this does not mean that we can do without movement or that movement does not add very real benefits.

Muscles in good condition pump blood more efficiently through blood vessels, thereby helping to prevent varicose veins and lymphedema of the legs. Well-conditioned muscles help prevent backaches; help us keep our bellies flatter and more comfortable; keep us strong for carrying books, briefcases, groceries, laundry, kids, and furniture; and help keep our skin in better condition. Because oxygen is carried more efficiently to these muscles, all work is easier, and we can continue any practiced movement for longer periods of time. We should remain capable of hard work and hard play.

All muscles work to help pump the blood back to the heart. Walking by itself is a powerful help to our circulation: the tightening of the muscles helps pump the blood very efficiently back up, against gravity, from the legs to the heart. Jogging presents some problems of its own.

Look seriously at jogging in relation to yourself — and the only body you'll ever have.

What happens to the breasts when the feet send wave after wave of impact up through the body as your feet meet the pavement? The larger and heavier the breasts, the more wear and tear on the tissue will result from their bouncing. Cone-shaped breasts will suffer more damage than the breasts with a wider base. The less support the brassiere gives, the more damage will be done. Even with good support, the pull of shoulder strap into soft flesh may cause numbness, tingling or pain in your hands, arms, shoulder, and neck. If you develop this problem, widen your shoulder straps significantly. Move the straps on your brassiere along your shoulder till they are away from an area that makes your arms tingle. *Never allow any tingling* or loss of feeling to continue. Change your arm position or the position of the straps, but stop the tingling.

The softer the surface you run on, the less damage will be done. The lighter you land, the less damage will be done. During menstrual periods and pregnancy, the tone of belly muscles and colon are down, and they, too, bounce more in jogging. If you develop or already have very strong belly muscles before you begin jogging, you should be able to jog safely. Many women find that they wet themselves while running, at least before menstruation. If you feel any dragging or pulling pain, you probably shouldn't jog at all; you certainly should do less jogging. To reverse the effects of gravity and impact shocks, after jogging or walking you should lie down and elevate your hips and legs several times a day.

In late pregnancy there is another factor to be taken into account — the loosening of pelvic ligaments because of natural hormonal action. Any pounding of feet against even a soft surface at this time may get you into trouble. Even the strongest hip and thigh muscles cannot prevent nature from taking its course and loosening the ligaments in the whole pelvic area.

This same hormonal loosening happens to some women with each menstrual period. The women who do have this loosening find it much easier to work for flexibility during their periods because the ligaments give so well. But it should be considered a danger signal for runners and jumpers.

Because of the greater pelvic angle in women, those who are even slightly overweight or have a tendency to knock-knees probably should not take up jogging unless they take great care to land lightly and run only on soft surfaces. Knee problems abound in people who jog, even among those of the right weight. Be sure, when you choose an activity, to choose one that will not damage you.

The same reasoning applies to the clothes you choose for jogging or exercise. Nothing you wear should stop blood flow or restrict movement of joints. Jersey sweatpants or loose shorts are best. Many underpants are too tight around the groin area. In the premenstrual and menstrual periods and during pregnancy, there is raised pressure in leg veins. A pair of underpants that digs in at the groin can restrict the return blood flow from the legs because the large veins lie just under the skin where the thigh joins the pelvis. This can cause pain, worsen varicose veins, or actually cause varicose veins. Even just sitting and standing in such pants can cause problems. Get rid of them or cut or loosen the elastic.

Women dancers and joggers, even many inactive women, find that the I.U.D. (intrauterine device) causes excessive bleeding. The loss of blood also lowers your iron and calcium levels.

The irritation, as you run, of tampon against vaginal walls can be a cause of backache. This is an individual sensitivity. Some women suffer from backaches when they use tampons even though they do not move very much.

With all of these considerations in mind, whether you should or shouldn't jog often comes down to whether you're "going to do it in spite of . . ."

How to Jog

If you're in good condition, jogging can be great all-around exercise, provided you *start slowly and work up gradually* to full, prolonged jogging. Here's how. Watch for problems. Never continue any exercise that causes you pain or other problems when done as directed. It's your body; protect it.

Start with walking, slowly at first. Draft a friend to walk along with you for a leisurely chat, or take the dog out for a restrained airing. Wear comfortable, light-weight clothes. Running shoes or sneakers are great.

Build up until you can easily walk a mile. Don't be in a hurry. Take your time. Enjoy yourself. Each day, walk just a little farther, until you reach a mile.

Speed up the walking. If you're walking a mile, now is the time to stretch your legs out and walk fast. Slow down immediately if you get short of breath, tired, or dizzy. These are not serious signs; they are caution signals from your body. Listen carefully to your body. Increase your speed again when caution signals ease. Each day you'll do better. Try to work up to a mile, walking faster the whole time. Take as long a period of time as you want — a week or two or three. Just be sure you *practice every day* for positive results!

Before beginning jogging, do some stretches and warm up your joints. *Walk fast and, every now and then, jog a few steps.* Again, listen to your body. Slow down at any caution signals. Don't push forward into jogging too fast. You have lots of time! *Build up the jogging each day until you can jog a mile.* You can, at this point, choose to speed up your jogging, or you can try jogging a little farther each day. No straining, ever! Don't stop suddenly! Taper off. Take the last five or ten minutes to slow down gradually. Walk it off.

Caution: If you stop running for a few days, go easy in distance and speed when you start again, and work up slowly.

EXERCISE BICYCLE

Bad weather, bad neighborhoods — any number of things may make it difficult to keep yourself in good physical condition by walking, jogging, or riding a regular bicycle. But you can find a good alternative. The exercise bike may be perfect for you. Use it at home, any time, for only as long as you want, in any clothes except those that bind. You can write on a clipboard, watch TV, or read as you ride. It is a real boon for those times when you can't do other exercises.

An exercise bike is useful in helping to improve endurance, circulation, and breathing, and is particularly beneficial for

- hard-working people who have great need but little time for exercise;
- those under stress who need to work off their tensions;
- those who live in cold climates or where the winters are long;
- those without easily accessible places to exercise;
- those who are at all unsure of their footing or their balance;
- those who live on strict time schedules;
- those who live where walking or jogging outside would be risky because of muggers or potholes;
- those who cannot put their whole body weight on their feet because of severe varicose veins or lymphedema;
- those with knee, foot, hip, or leg problems that are not made worse with use of the exercise bike (rule of thumb: if it hurts, don't do it!);
- those with high blood pressure;
- the obese, who may injure hip, knee, or foot joints when running or even walking.

How to Choose an Exercise Bike

Look for one that

- was built to be a stationary bike, not one with a converted base that was originally meant to be a regular bike;
- has no motor, because you supply the energy;
- has a base sufficiently sturdy so there's no rocking when you get on or off or while you're riding, no matter how fast or how hard you push;

- has a padded seat that can be adjusted for height;
- has adjustable handlebars;
- has straps to hold your feet on the pedals;
- has a chain guard to keep your clothing from getting caught;
- has a pressure adjustment to allow you gradually to increase the strength you need for pedaling.

Mile and minute meters are all right, but not necessary. And you may want to add a lamb's-wool seat cover for added comfort.

How to Use the Bike

- Start with the pressure knob at lowest possible level.
- The first day, ride well within the limits where you feel comfortable, even if that means pushing the pedals only four or five times. Don't do more.
- The second day, repeat the same amount, but do it twice, once in the morning and once in the evening.
- The third day, if you still feel no ill effects, do the same routine three times.
- Stay at this level for several days or until you feel that you can comfortably add a little more time.

In the beginning, be extremely cautious and add very small amounts of extra time. Do not increase the pedaling to the point where you are breathing *very* hard. A little harder is fine. As you continue building slowly over the first month, you will begin to develop a feeling as to how your body is reacting to the little extra work each day.

You will find as you continue that you can increase, both in time and in speed, at a slightly faster rate. Don't push it too fast, but work up to the point where you are riding rapidly — not full tilt, but rapidly — for an hour at a time or three twenty-minute periods a day. Try reading or watching TV to avoid boredom. Now begin to turn the knob that increases the pressure on the wheel, increasing it very slightly. Judge for yourself how much you can do and develop the program for yourself accordingly, making it harder or faster or both.

With a sensible approach, you should be able to do yourself an incredible amount of good in a very cautious manner.

Problems the Exercise Bike Can Help

Circulatory problems: First ride the bike slowly, *using no added pressure on the wheel.* If you have lymphedema or varicose veins, do not try to reach great speeds too rapidly; the delicacy of the tissues and blood vessels can cause them to be damaged if you force speed or pressure. If your lower legs have been discolored, swollen, or ulcerated, take a good long while before you add extra pressure, and then add it very gradually. Add no extra pressure till the color of the legs is much improved, even if it takes months.

Obesity: Since even walking, when you are overweight, is a strain on the heart, work more for circulation than for strength. This means that, with no turning of the pressure knob at all, you slowly increase the amount of time you can spend on the bike, working only to the point where your breathing is increased a little. Many overweight people have high blood pressure. It is wise to keep the degree of progression low while still continuing to progress. Since your joints are not built to carry a lot of extra weight steadily, using an exercise bike is excellent and should be a basic exercise for anyone who is overweight by twenty-five pounds or more. If you can't afford to buy your own bike, find one to use at a local YWCA or health club.

Breathing problems: When breathing problems are really serious, the muscles are not getting enough oxygen for them to be able to work strongly or very long. This forms a vicious circle. Again, it means you must work for a very gradual buildup, but *never* to the point of exhaustion. Excessive work can, in fact, do more harm than good. An exercise bike is excellent for those of you with breathing problems because it keeps you close to your rest areas.

Balance problems: People with balance problems can be separated into two groups: those who with increased endurance will regain their balance, and those who have more permanent problems and possibly may not regain their balance.

The first group should eventually be able to leave the bike and go on to other means of exercise. People with permanent loss of balance will probably need the bike for maintaining endurance, circulation, and breathing for the rest of their lives, although they should also walk and continue a normal life in other ways. Although the walking may not be of a quality that can add significantly to their physical health, it is important for their emotional well-being.

13

Balance and Dizziness

The feeling that you're turning around or that things are turning around you is a condition that makes you lose your balance. It can happen for all sorts of reasons — a disease of the inner ear; unbalanced electrolytes or certain other changes in the blood and lymph; injury to the semicircular canals in the inner ear caused by your turning around too fast and too long (which is why ballerinas "spot" when they pirouette); low blood pressure; limb muscles too weak to control the flow of blood smoothly when you shift position; or many over-the-counter or prescription drugs such as antihistamines. All or any of these can make you dizzy or cause vertigo and loss of balance. Anemia, low blood sugar, long periods of time spent without moving, changes in weight, any sickness or stress, or a host of other conditions can affect your sense of balance — sometimes very badly. To regain balance in spite of dizziness takes practice as well as therapy.

EMERGENCY MEASURES

Your body has the least trouble adjusting to gravity when you are lying down, completely supported. As an emergency measure when you're on your feet — if you get dizzy or feel "pitched" and feel you're going to fall — grab hold of something sturdy nearby and stoop, crouch, kneel, or sit. The important thing is to *lower* your center of

Figure 1

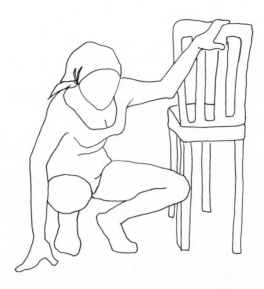

gravity. (See Figure 1.) This will make it less likely that you will fall and possibly hurt yourself. If you're *very* dizzy, *lie down!*

The whole body is always involved in the attempt to balance. Look at a baby when he or she first starts to walk. Look at what the baby does in a year — in ten years — with practice. Some type of balance is a part of every activity because the organ of balance, the vestibular system, controls all our reflexes, the movements of our eyes, and even our viscera, as happens in motion sickness. You become suddenly consciously aware of a *lack* of balance when you feel queasy from air- or seasickness, when you feel dizzy, very weak, feel "pitched," as with vertigo, or have a fear of falling.

If you have problems with balance, there just isn't any substitute for practicing until you can move well, or at least better. You become good at what you practice — and practice — and practice. Acrobats, astronauts, ballerinas, and others all get practice in doing unusual things to achieve balance and combat dizziness.

LEARNING TO ACCOMMODATE

Dizziness, sometimes even vertigo, which makes you feel as if you're pitching over, can be handled often by accommodation — by getting used to it or learning how to operate in spite of it. If you let dizziness

Figure 2

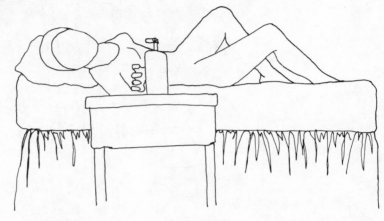

prevent your moving, you may never get around to moving. This is how you approach working toward an accommodation. Start where you feel safest, lying in bed though dizzy. Have some objects that will not break easily, maybe small cans of food, on tables at either side of the bed. Turn your head slowly toward one table, then reach out and try to grab one of the cans, making sure to keep your eyes on it till you finally connect. (See Figure 2.) Do the same on the other side. It is a good idea to limit your first attempts at accommodation to a few minutes. And practice only after an hour or so following a meal, since most people become nauseated when they get dizzy.

Caution: If turning your head makes you dizzier and nauseated, and these feelings continue after the practice session for more than ten minutes, try the exercise more slowly. If all else fails, turn your eyes instead of your head.

LEARNING TO TURN

Next, move to an armchair — a good, sturdy armchair. (Sit in front of a sturdy kitchen table to prevent your tipping onto the floor.) With a small table on either side of the chair, again place a can on either side of you.

This is important! Grab hold of both arms of the chair if you are dizzy. Now, letting go of *only one arm of the chair,* turn your head or your eyes toward one of the tables. (See Figure 3.) Reach with one hand to pick up the can, and then transfer it to the table on the other side. If you suffer from vertigo, judge the rate of speed at which you can turn without pitching. Practice that timing till you can repeat it every time.

Now, still keeping hold of the chair, turn your eyes or your head to the other side and try for the can with the other hand. The timing or rate of speed at which you can turn your head to avoid dizziness may be different for each side. Practice every day, several times a day, till you can grab the can every time and have perfected the timing so as not to increase your dizziness or vertigo.

Next, try picking up the can from the table in front of you. When you feel more sure of yourself, try picking up the can from the floor from different spots. Again, try reaching for the can without holding on to the chair arm only when you feel totally sure of yourself. (See

Figure 3

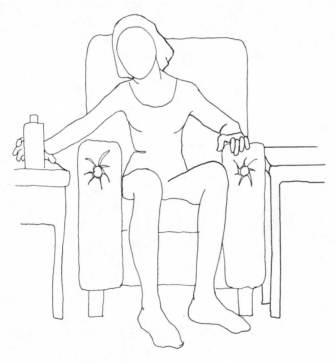

Figure 4.) Have someone else put the cans around you and feel the difference when you reach for them. (See Figure 5.)

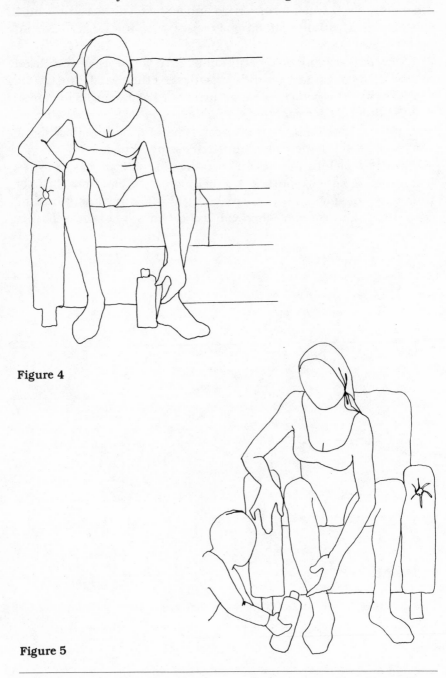

Figure 4

Figure 5

Don't begin the next step until you're completely ready for it.

This time, start with an overstuffed armchair behind you so that you'll sit in it if you fall. Stand behind a sturdy chair. Hold on and walk in place. (See Figure 6.) If this doesn't bother you at all, or when it finally doesn't, try turning your head very slowly from side to side and continue walking. Get a little more courageous, as you become accustomed to moving while dizzy, and try turning your head slowly and then nodding your head slowly — and continue to walk in place, still holding on to the chair. Also try pivoting (slowly at first till you find the correct rate of speed) to the left and pivoting to the right. Pivoting the body may work for some who cannot turn only their heads without becoming dizzy.

Figure 6

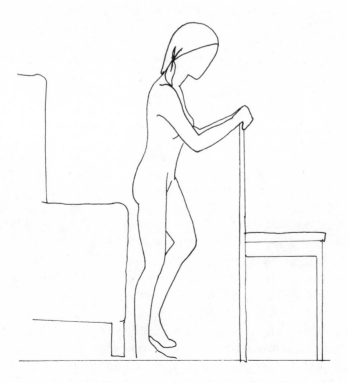

Figure 7

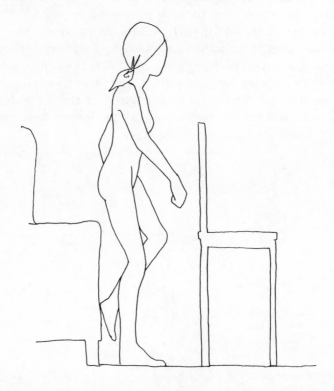

When you feel completely able to, try walking in place without holding on but with both chairs still in place for reassurance. (See Figure 7.) If possible, begin cautiously and slowly to nod and turn your head. At the same time, initiate the normal swinging of your arms at your sides in time to your feet. (See Figure 8.) Many people learn to handle dizziness but walk the rest of their lives as if they expect to fall — arms out a little to the sides, elbows bent, and hands ready to grab something or to protect them if they fall forward. If you feel very unsure of your balance, use a cane or a walker. Always use a banister when walking up or down stairs if you tend to get dizzy, and certainly hold on to banisters always if you suffer from vertigo. (See Figure 9.) If you can manage without the cane or walker, use your arms as normally as possible. The swing of your arms helps your balance. Let them swing. Practice it.

Figure 8

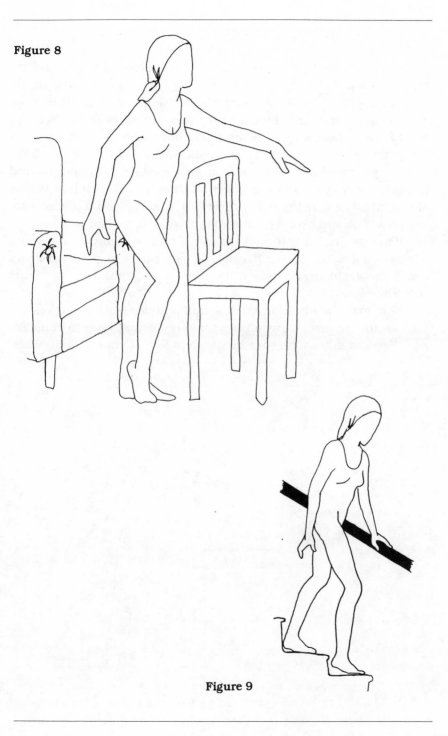

Figure 9

PRACTICING YOUR BALANCING ACT

The next step is to practice your new balancing act in a less re-
stricted area. Pull a sturdy kitchen table out into the center of the
room or use the desk. Now, with one hand on the desk or table, start
walking around it. (See Figure 10.) When you're ready, try to begin
nodding your head a little. When you're handling that well, try turning your head and continue to walk around the table or desk.
Change your walking direction from time to time. Some people find
it much easier to turn in one direction than the other. If that is true
of you, practice turning in the direction in which you feel least sure
of yourself till you become somewhat more accustomed to it.

When you're ready to try your wings solo — no props — be sure
to start on a well-carpeted floor if you can. Slippery or waxed floors
should not be in any home or office. Remember the old saying "Pride
cometh before a fall"?

Now you're ready to practice — and practice is what it takes. No
one retains the use of any ability that she doesn't keep in constant
use. Become a busy person; be on your feet as much as possible.

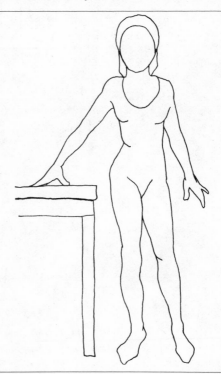

Figure 10

The more you move, the less you will tend to notice your dizziness (unless you are consciously trying to or don't have enough to do to keep you diverted). Of course, abrupt changes in the extent of dizziness, such as you will get if you have vertigo, will always call themselves to your attention. Don't sneeze! It may take you a few minutes every day to become accustomed to going in one direction while your head seems to be going in the other. The more you use your hands, the better your judgment of where to reach for something will become. Again, it will take constant and regular practice.

Never again use bifocals. They will give you more trouble with balance. Two pairs of glasses are going to be best for you.

Check your diet, as suggested earlier. Make it the kind of diet suitable for you. Diet *can* be all-important. Check out every possibility, with your doctor's help.

But even though you're dizzy, live actively and you will live better, even if you must do all exercises lying on your back. Movement is necessary to keep the rest of the body functioning well.

Don't ever, under any circumstances, pretend to be dizzier than you are for someone else's benefit. You have to convince yourself to convince them. Acting dizzy is going to lose you the battle you're out to win. But treat dizziness as you would pain. If you've got to live with it, you should try to move in spite of it.

DIZZINESS ON GETTING UP SUDDENLY

Dizziness that occurs when you get out of bed or up from the floor, or when you rise too quickly from a leaning-over position, occurs because your brain becomes anemic. The blood tends to move to the lower parts of the body until the muscles in your legs become active and shove the blood from the veins back to your heart rapidly enough and the vascular reflexes begin to work. That is why it is important to increase the muscle tone in your legs before rising, and to rise slowly. Although dizziness is common in older people, even young active people will faint if they are strapped to a table and suddenly tilted upright.

But there is another factor at work. In your neck you have measuring devices on the two carotid arteries that carry blood to the brain. They read the pressure in the arteries and then readjust the blood pressure so that the pressure in the circulation to the head is neither too low nor too high. In some people, this sort of measuring element is apparently oversensitive and responds to tight collars, sudden head movements, and the like by dropping blood pressure strongly. In others, the reflex is too slow; when you change your position, there is a time lag before the blood pressure readjusts. This is particularly true in older people.

If you get dizzy when you get up suddenly, don't try to ignore it or think that you can overcome it by medication. Instead, learn how to deal with it by finding the best ways of changing posture without getting dizzy, and then practice those ways until they become a habit. (If these methods do not work, and you continue to be dizzy often, see your doctor.)

The following is a useful procedure for two reasons. First, it slows down the act of getting up from a lying-down posture. Second, it "pumps up" your muscle tone so as to combat the drop in blood pressure that occurs when you stand up.

While lying in bed, do the following "tightening" movements. Do them hard, and in order. (See Figure 11.)

- Clench your toes.
- Pull your toes toward your knees.
- Pull your thighs hard in against each other.
- Clench all the muscles in your bottom.
- Tighten your belly by bearing down hard against the bed.
- Tighten your shoulders, arms, and hands by pushing your hands in against each other.
- Tighten your neck by pulling your head up and jaw forward.
- Tighten your face by pursing your mouth and squeezing your eyes tight shut.

Figure 11

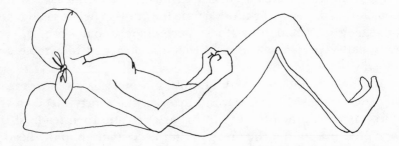

Now! Relax completely: flop your arms and legs, roll your head, and blop your belly in and out. (See Figure 12.) And then stretch right arm up, right leg down, then left arm up, left leg down. (See Figure 13.)

Breathe deeply a couple of times, and then slowly push yourself up on one elbow, then up to a sitting posture, and finally slowly get up on your feet. (See Figure 14.)

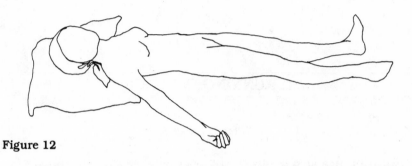

Figure 12

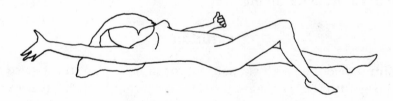

Figure 13

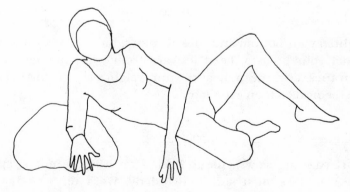

Figure 14

14
The Twenty Most Important Exercises

---

1. RUNNING IN PLACE

What It Does

Running in place is one of the best all-around warm-up exercises. Running pushes blood faster, warms up the body, and starts adrenalin running.

Caution

Run barefoot on a thick, soft mat or in soft-soled, thick-soled shoes, with the least noise possible. Keep your back flat. (Check it against a wall.) Start slowly and then slow down gradually.

Position

Tighten your bottom and tuck it under, hard. Cross your arms under your breasts. Lean forward from your hips with your chin tucked in. Keep most of your weight on your big toe and the toe next to it on each foot.

Exercise

Start running slowly, toe to heel. After a few minutes, speed up. Your feet must still land quietly. Work up over days to running as fast as you can, always after the slow beginning. Remember to slow down gradually.

How Long

Work up to one minute slowly, and increase the tempo as necessary. Increase the amount of time gradually to three minutes to five minutes to eight minutes.

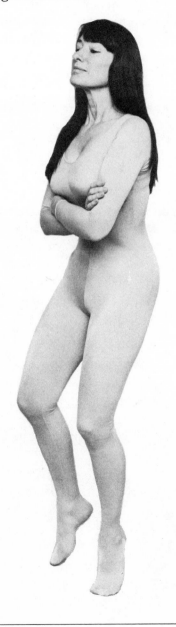

2. BICYCLE EXERCISE

What It Does

This exercise is excellent for all of the belly muscles and the neck, and even gives some reasonably good exercise to the front of the thighs, inner and outer thighs, and the hips.

Position

Lie on your back, either on your bed if it is firm or on a rug or mat on the floor. Lift your head and tuck your chin into your chest. Bring both knees up to your chest.

Exercise

Straighten out one leg, pointing upward, so that it is over the hip on that side; then bring it back down to the chest. Do the same with the other leg. This is the bicycle exercise. Now lower both legs, keeping the back of your waistline on the floor or bed. Lower your legs just a little bit more every day, as far as you can without letting your back arch up. Never let your legs go lower than about five or six inches from the floor. Your waistline must remain on the floor to tighten your belly muscles properly.

For the side waistline, roll over onto one side and prop yourself up on your elbow. Continue to do the same bicycling exercise. When you're tired, roll over onto the other side and do the exercise the same number of times. When you can, after several days or weeks, keep your arms folded in front of you as you bicycle.

Caution

Keep your chin tucked in close!

How Many

Do ten repetitions in each of the three positions — on your back and on your right and left sides. Work up gradually to fifty repetitions a day, done in sets of ten. If you have serious problems with your belly, four to six sets of fifty repetitions a day are worth working up to. This is a great TV commercial–break exercise.

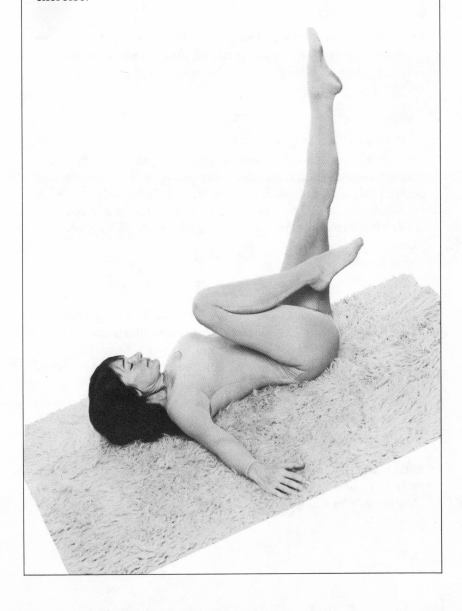

3. WAISTLINE PULL

What It Does

This exercise is for pulling in your belly muscles and forming a better waistline. It tightens up the front diaphragm.

Caution

Proceed very slowly if you have a hiatus hernia. If the exercise makes you dizzy, pull in less or hold your breath for a shorter period of time. It is best done on an empty stomach.

Position

Do belly bloppers to prepare for this exercise. Then stand with your feet apart, knees bent, fingers turned in, and hands braced on your thighs just above your knees. Curl your pelvis under. Inhale as much as possible; exhale completely. With breath still exhaled pull your belly in and up under your rib cage. Hold the position for just a second. Relax and breathe normally.

Attention

After you've exhaled, if you close up the back of your throat to make a "kh" sound, you can force more air out and make more room for the next step, which is pulling your belly way in as far as you can and way up underneath your rib cage. After your first effort at pulling in, pull in even more.

If you pull your hands back against your bent knees as you pull in your belly, you will be able to get your belly in much farther, contracting the muscles more.

As you get better at pulling in, the muscles will get more and more efficient and you will begin to see that the muscles, as they tighten, can pull you in at the back of your waistline also. (Check in the mirror.)

How Many

This exercise takes several days to several weeks to perform properly. Within six weeks you can usually take an inch to an inch and a half off your waistline by doing the exercise to the best of your ability ten times a day.

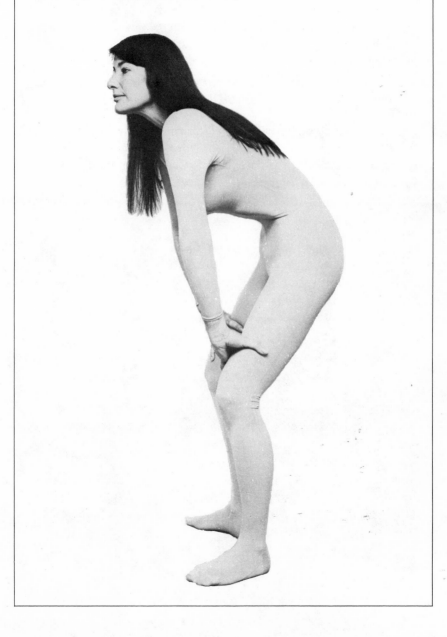

4. CROSSOVER ABDOMINAL EXERCISE

What It Does

This exercise is wonderful for your waistline, is especially good for the side abdominals, and is good for flexibility of the back. It is also good for pulling the rib cage back into place after pregnancy.

Position

Lie on your back on your bed, if it is firm, or on a rug or mat on the floor. Lift your head and tuck your chin into your chest. Bring both knees up to your chest. Clasp your hands behind your head.

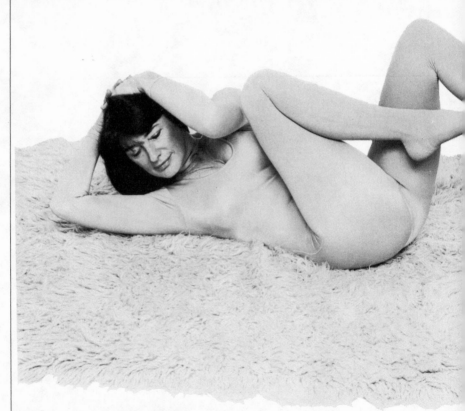

Exercise

Twist your shoulders and legs to bring one knee to the outside of the opposite shoulder. Then do the same with the other knee and its opposite shoulder. Continue alternating as long as you can.

Attention

As you get stronger, try to pull the knees up a little closer by lifting the shoulders up a little farther off the ground.

How Many

Work your way up to fifty, in sets of ten done five times a day. Then, if you need more work on side abdominals, gradually build up to two to four sets of fifty repetitions a day.

5. BACK-OF-WAIST TRIMMER

What It Does

This exercise is for the outer sides of the long and short muscles of the back. It is also good for side-to-side flexibility of the body.

Position

Stand with your legs and feet apart, farther than width of your hips. Turn your feet in slightly. Press down hard with the big toe and the one next to it. Lean forward slightly and tuck your bottom under so that your back is flat. Bend your fists up to your shoulders.

Exercise

Pull your right hip forward as you pull your right elbow back. Pull your left hip forward as you pull your left elbow back.

Attention

Get into a rhythm and continue at a nice steady pace.

How Many

Work up to twenty-five repetitions; then gradually up to fifty repetitions. If your whole midsection at the back needs a lot of help, work up gradually to fifty repetitions three to six times a day.

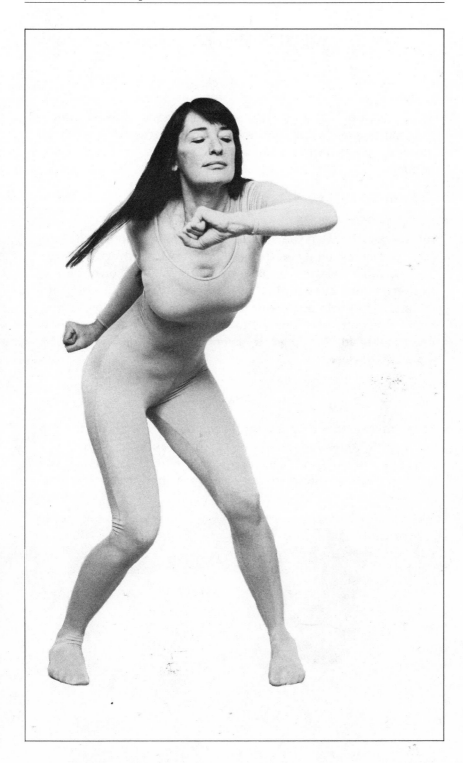

6. BOTTOM CLENCHER

What It Does

If you are out of shape, this exercise can take from two and a half to three and a half inches off the outer upper thighs (when measured together) and can lift the buttocks from one to two inches.

Position

Lie on your back on the floor or bed. Bend your knees slightly. Let your knees hang out. Support your upper body with pillows so that your waistline is pressed gently to the floor or bed. If you are strong enough, lift your head and tuck your chin into your chest to help push your waistline down to the floor. If you can't hold your head up, put pillows behind your upper shoulders and head. For the entire exercise, your waistline must be against the floor.

Exercise

Now put one foot over the top of the other. Push with the top foot while you pull with the lower. Tighten your buttocks as hard as you can, and use the pressure of one foot against the other to help you keep them tight. Don't just hold them tight,

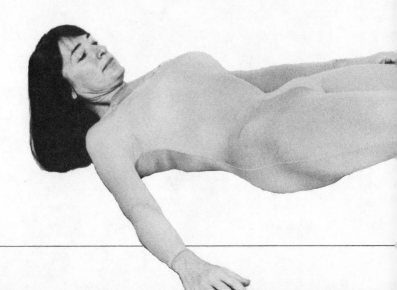

but continue to retighten them more every few seconds. Switch foot positions and repeat.

Attention

As you become able to keep your waistline down more easily, start removing pillows from behind your head and shoulders. You should, at the same time, be practicing so that you can keep your chin as close to your chest as possible throughout the entire exercise.

When you can keep your head up, chin tucked into your chest, and have no pillows behind your shoulders, try extending your legs little by little, always being sure to keep the knees slightly bent.

See if with time you can hold your buttocks rock-hard for a full ten minutes a day — maybe for two minutes at a time.

Practicing keeping the buttocks tight as you move can be a positive, long-term help. A good habit.

Caution

When your knees are completely straight, your back arches, and this can cause back problems.

How Many

Start gradually with one or two spaced over a day. As your strength increases daily, try to hold the muscles tighter and for a longer period of time. Most women with prominent saddle-bags can lose two and a half to three inches in six weeks by holding this position for an accumulated ten minutes a day.

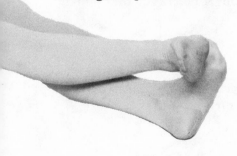

7. UPPER-HIP EXERCISE

What It Does

This exercise is excellent for the upper part of the hip and lower part of your waistline in the back. These tend to start turning to flab by the time we reach our early twenties.

Position

Facing the foot of the bed, sit on the right edge with your left knee folded up on the bed in front of you. Stretch the right leg out behind you to touch the floor. Rest your arms, elbow to hand, on the left side beyond the folded leg.

Exercise

Lean over far enough so that you can lift the right leg up with the knee bent behind you as far back as possible and swing the knee forward and back. Try five to ten swings as far forward and as far back as you can get. Now straighten the leg and continue to swing it forward and back.

Attention

Leaning forward more will help you get your leg off the ground, but once you can get it up more easily, bring yourself farther upright by rising up higher on your hands. This way, you will get the muscles at the back of the waistline contracted more. (This is usually difficult to achieve when you first begin. If necessary, wait until you are stronger before you lift up higher on your hands.)

How Many

Work your way up to two or three sets of ten repetitions each day and finally thirty repetitions on each side at one sitting.

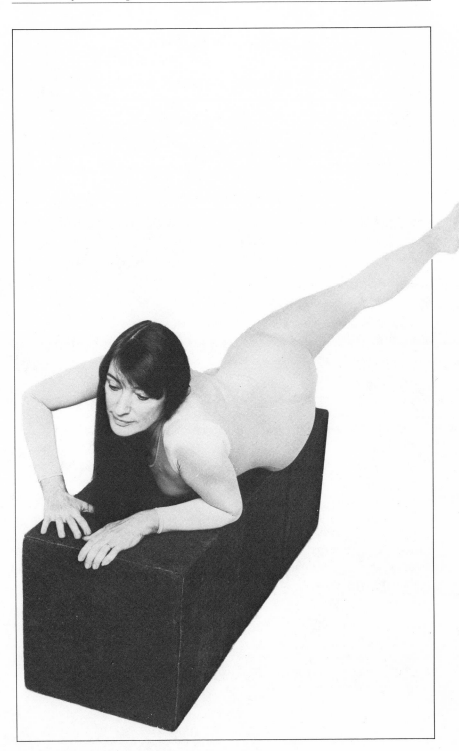

8. THIGH TONER

What It Does

Well-developed thigh muscles hold your kneecaps in place, lift you up and down, and give you nicely shaped, firm thighs.

Attention

You really must do this exercise or ride an exercise bike for at least fifteen minutes a day with gradually increasing pressure. Be sure to "oil" the knees before beginning the exercise. (See page 57.)

Position

Stand with your back flat against a wall, your knees bent, and bare feet about a foot and a half apart and about six to eight inches out from the wall.

Exercise

Be sure to keep your back flat to the wall. Make sure that you can look down and see three toes of each foot inside your knee. Bend your knees a little more till you feel the muscles of your thighs contract. Hold the position for about thirty seconds or as long as you can or bounce gently in that position. Slide down the wall a little farther and repeat. Continue to slide down as far as you can or until you're squatting.

Lean forward over your feet with your head dropped forward and bounce gently several times. If you can, or when you can (maybe in three weeks or so), return up the wall the same way, keeping your back flat to the wall the whole way.

Caution

Remember to keep your knees placed so that you can see some of your toes between your knees.

How Many

Begin by doing this exercise once at three well-separated times each day. Later, you can add on as you feel able to till you can do eight to ten slow repetitions daily.

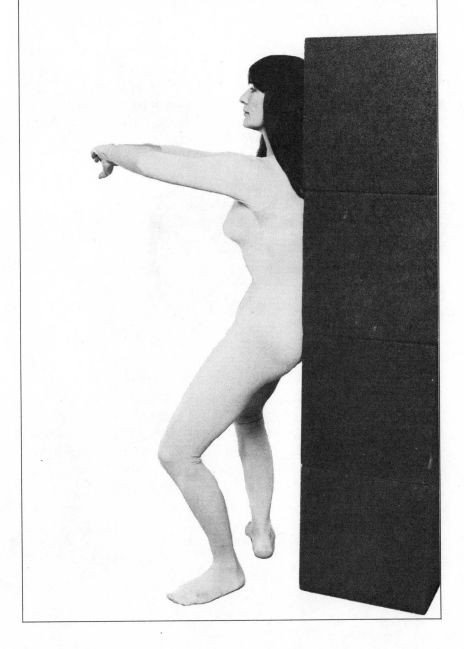

9. INNER-THIGH EXERCISE I

What It Does

This is one way to exercise the inner thighs.

Position

Sit on the floor, leaning to the left side on your left hand with the right arm across your belly. Bend your right knee with your foot placed firmly on the floor. Bring the left leg out straight in front. Make sure your back is not arching. Turn your left foot out so that the arch is toward the ceiling.

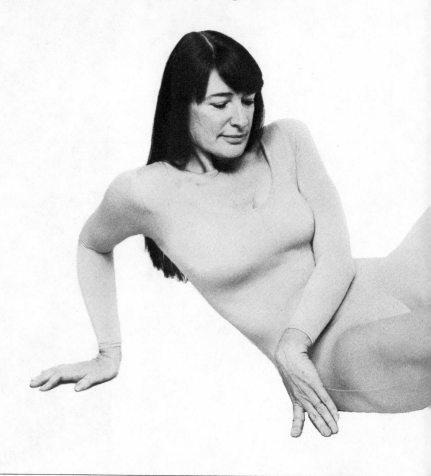

Exercise

Lift and lower the raised left leg. Continue to lift and lower the leg as you bring the leg a little farther out to the side till it is as close to the shoulder as you can get it. Exercise the right leg the same way.

Attention

Try to keep the leg as straight as possible without letting the knee lock. Keep the foot turned out, and keep the back from arching.

How Many

These exercises will be tiring in the beginning. Work your way up to at least twenty-five a day for each leg.

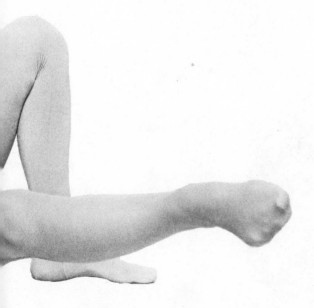

10. INNER-THIGH EXERCISE II

What It Does

This exercise also helps the inner thighs.

Position

Lie on your back on the floor with your feet up the wall. Keep your knees bent and almost together and turn your toes way in. Keep your head down on the floor and your chin tucked into your chest.

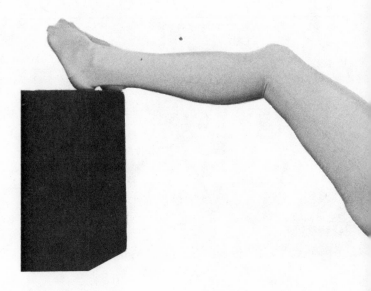

Exercise

Tighten your buttocks and your inner thighs to lift your bottom slowly off the floor. Lift your bottom only. Keep your waistline down. Now lower your bottom and raise and lower it many times.

Attention

This exercise need not be done at all if you are using a bike, stationary or otherwise, for a half-hour a day — *Regularly!*

How Many

You can't do too many.

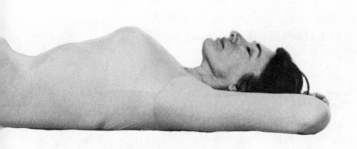

11. BEAUTIFUL-CALF EXERCISE

What It Does

It will be obvious from the way your legs ache after you first start that these toe rises are good for your calves. Pressing in your big toe and the one next to it will also develop your arch very strongly, especially if the exercise is continued over a long period of time.

Position

Stand with your feet turned slightly out under your hips, knees just slightly unlocked. Hold on to a sink or bureau if you need to for balance.

Exercise

Come as high up onto your big toe and the one next to it as possible, pressing your toes hard into the floor. Tighten up at the back of your heels by pushing the front of your foot forward as hard as you can.

Stand on your right foot with the toes of your left foot behind your right calf. Come up onto the toes of the right foot. Do an equal number of times on each foot.

Attention

If one calf is smaller than the other, repeat the exercise more often on the smaller side till the calves are symmetrical.

How Many

Starting with three sets of ten several times a day, gradually work your way up to doing thirty at one time. When it is easy to do about thirty of these toe rises, try them standing on one leg at a time, thirty on each side.

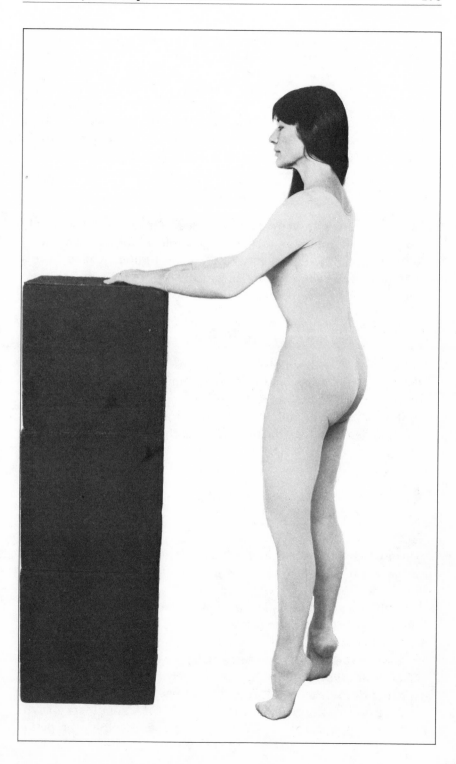

12. UPPER-BODY STRAIGHTENER

What It Does

This exercise unrounds your shoulders. It stretches out the front of your chest and tightens up the muscles across the upper back. It is excellent for upper-body posture.

Position

Sit in a chair with your feet apart, lean forward slightly, and get your back to feel as arched as possible. (Your back will not actually be arched. The muscles will be tightened down the length of your back. As long as your knees are bent in front of you, your back cannot arch.) Keep your chin level

Attention

(To get a feel for how the exercise moves your shoulder, try this first: put one hand on the opposite shoulder while the arm hangs at your side, thumb turned in. With thumb turning up and back, roll your shoulder as you bring your straight arm up to shoulder level, out to the side, and then back as far as you can.)

Hunch up your shoulders and pull them down as far as possible.

Exercise

Now, with both arms hanging, thumbs turned in, bring both arms up in front of you to shoulder level, thumbs facing each other and out to the side and back as far as you can with thumbs turning out as far as possible. Make sure your shoulders roll back. Watch the movement of your shoulders in a mirror.

Work the muscles harder: bend your elbows slightly, make fists, and tense up the arms completely. Now keep your arms tense. Lift and roll your arms, shoulders, and thumbs back in a rhythmic fashion. Inhale as you roll your shoulders back; exhale as you roll them forward. After a few swinging repetitions, keep your arms as far back as you can and bounce your tensed arms up and down a few inches.

How Many

Work your way up gradually to twenty-five repetitions a day. If the swinging movement bothers your shoulders, after a few times just keep your thumbs back and, with your upper back and fists tight, use a tension bounce (a few inches up and down). Work up gradually to fifty bouncing repetitions if your shoulders are round. Then fifty bouncing repetitions several times a day if you still need more.

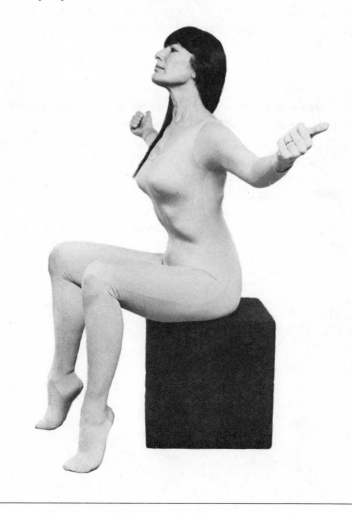

13. SPINE STRAIGHTENER

What It Does

This exercise is marvelous for posture; it will help you have a smooth and strong center back. It will also lift your chest and contract the long muscles that lie on either side of your spine down all the length of your back.

Caution

If you can't stretch your arms up, lie on your back, knees bent, arms at your sides. Slide them along the floor until they are overhead and press them against the floor.

Position

Sit in a chair with your feet apart, lean forward slightly, and get your back to feel as arched as possible. (Your back will not actually be arched. The muscles will be tightened down the length of your back. As long as your knees are bent in front of you, your back cannot arch.) Keep your chin level.

Take hold of one thumb with the other hand and stretch your arms straight up overhead along your ears. Keep your elbows very slightly bent and keep your back feeling arched. Hunch up your shoulders and bring them down as far as possible.

Exercise

Bounce your arms back from the shoulders over and over, arms still tensed, back still feeling arched.

Attention

Tighten the muscles of your arms and back a little more each day before you begin.

How Many

Work up gradually to fifty times a day.

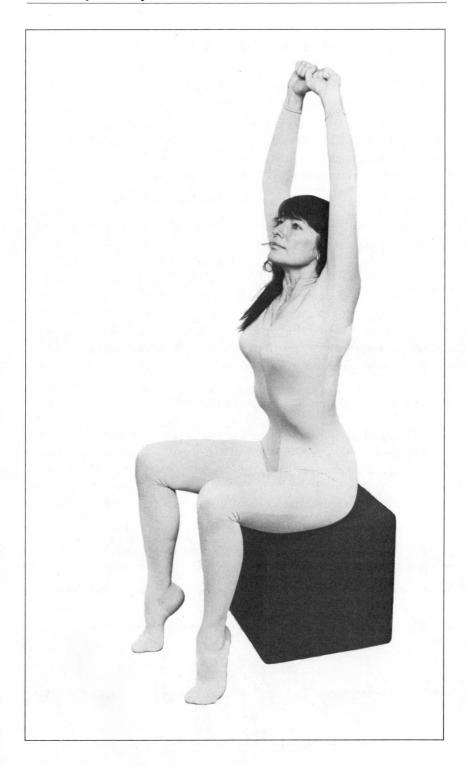

14. NECK STRAIGHTENER

What It Does

This exercise works the muscles from the base of the skull out to the shoulders and down to the mid and upper back just below the shoulder blades.

Position

Sit in a chair with your feet apart, lean forward slightly, and get your back to feel as arched as possible. (Your back will not actually be arched. The muscles will be tightened down the length of your back. As long as your knees are bent in front of you, your back cannot arch.) Keep your chin tucked in.

Clasp your hands behind your head. Do not arch your neck! Check to see that your shoulders are down by hunching up your shoulders and then letting them down. Keep your elbows back.

Exercise

Pull your hands against your head and push your head against your hands to tense all the muscles through the upper shoulders. Continue as far to one side as you can, pulling and resisting as you turn. Then do the same to the other side. Keep your eyes on the elbow that is moving back as you shift your head from side to side.

Attention

Each day try to pull with your hands and resist with your head a little more. Each day try to turn your elbows back a little farther. Keep breathing easily. Don't hold your breath.

How Many

You will never need more than twenty repetitions a day, ten for each side.

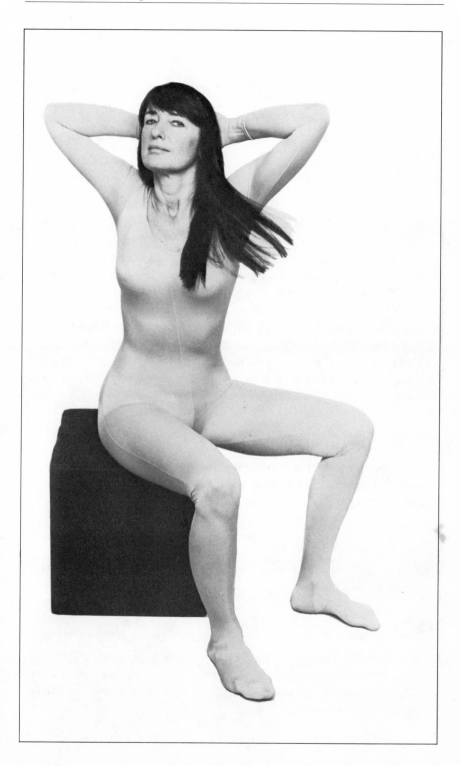

15. SHOULDER-BLADE FLATTENER

What It Does

This exercise strengthens the muscle that holds the shoulder blades firmly in place and keeps the sides of your rib cage smooth.

Position

Sit in a chair with your feet apart, lean forward slightly, and get your back to feel as arched as possible. (Your back will not actually be arched. The muscles will be tightened down the length of your back. As long as your knees are bent in front of you, your back cannot arch.) Keep your chin level.

Bend your elbows so that they are straight out from the shoulders, one thumb resting on each shoulder. Keep the elbows level with the shoulders throughout the entire exercise. Make a fist and tense your arms; hunch up your shoulders and bring them all the way down. Tighten up your whole upper back.

Exercise

Keep your arms and back tense as you turn your elbows and upper body as far back, side to side, as you can. Keep breathing and keep your head level and still.

Attention

Cautiously put a little more into the exercise each day. Tighten the muscle a little more. Turn a little farther.

How Many

Work up from ten repetitions three times a day to thirty at one time. If your upper back is very rounded or your shoulder blades are winging out (even a little), you need more. Try thirty repetitions three times a day.

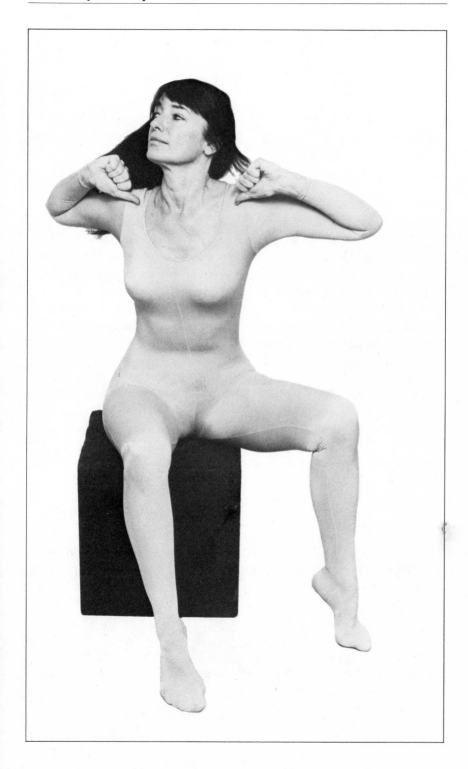

16. PECTORAL PUNCH

What It Does

This exercise is for the muscles across the chest, underlying the breasts, and also the arm muscles. It will help to keep your breasts from sagging.

Position

Sit in a chair with your feet apart, lean forward slightly, and get your back to feel as arched as possible. (Your back will not actually be arched. The muscles will be tightened down the length of your back. As long as your knees are bent in front of you, your back cannot arch.) Keep your chin level.

Bring your arms out in front of you just below armpit level and bend your elbows. Hunch up your shoulders and bring them down as far as possible.

Exercise

Make your hands into fists, one above the other, elbows kept high. Tighten up your arms and punch your arms across each other in front of you about four or five inches toward the opposite elbow, time after time.

Attention

Keep your elbows high. Exchange the position of your hands for the second half of the count, or just alternate as you punch. Increase the amount of tension in your arms as much as you can each day. You can always tighten up more than you think you can.

How Many

Work your way up to fifty repetitions; then, if you like, do fifty repetitions several times a day.

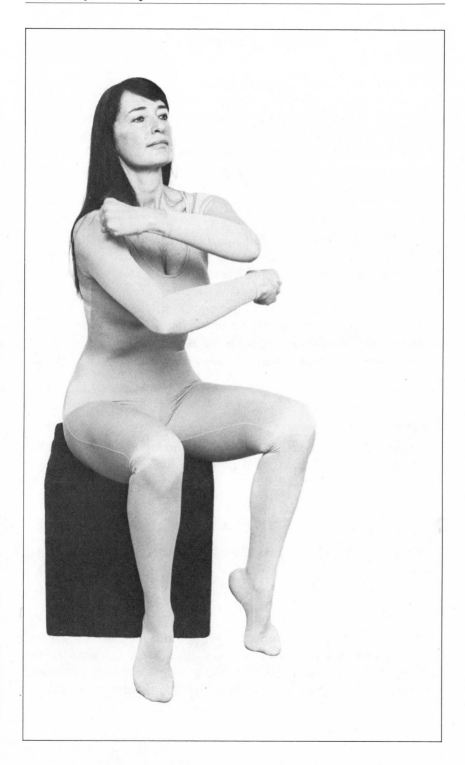

17. UNDERARM PRESS

What It Does

This exercise will help to tighten those muscles which make a loose, sloppy bulge high up on your back to the side, above and underneath the bra strap. Sometimes this is fat, but many times this bulge is underdeveloped muscle.

Position

Sit in a chair with your feet apart, lean forward slightly, and get your back to feel as arched as possible. (Your back will not actually be arched. The muscles will be tightened down the length of your back. As long as your knees are bent in front of you, your back cannot arch.) Keep your chin level.

Bend your elbows slightly and raise your arms to about waist level so that they make a big half circle in front of you. Keep your fists about twelve inches apart, thumbs toward you.

Exercise

Tense all your muscles through your arms and upper back. Bring your arms down, as if pressing against a great weight, all the way to your sides.

Attention

Each day try to tighten your muscles more as you do the exercise.

How Many

According to how your muscles are set in, how loose they tend to be, you may need more or less. Start with ten repetitions three times a day till you can do thirty once a day. If you need more, work up gradually to thirty repetitions three times a day.

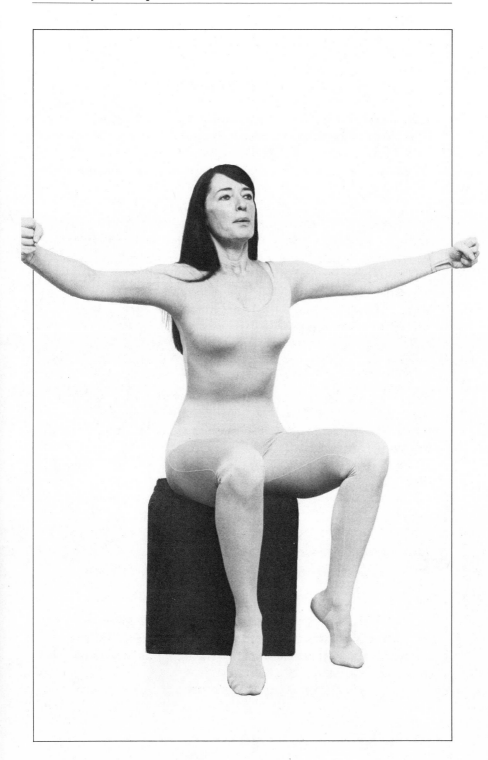

18. TOWEL TWIST

What It Does

This exercise does a beautiful job of developing muscles over your entire upper body and your arms.

Position

Sit in a chair with your feet apart, lean forward slightly, and get your back to feel as arched as possible. (Your back will not actually be arched. The muscles will be tightened down the length of your back. As long as your knees are bent in front of you, your back cannot arch.) Keep your chin level.

Take a very old towel, one you won't fret about if it's ruined, and lift it up to shoulder level as if you are going to wring it out. Keep your elbows high.

Exercise

Wring the towel as hard as you can in one direction so that you tighten all the way down the arms into the chest muscles and upper back muscles until the muscles tremble with the effort. Keep breathing regularly!

Now reverse the twist and let the other arm do the wringing.

Attention

Try to wring the towel harder each day.

How Many

Do this exercise three times a day on each side. Wring the towel as hard as you can and hold for a few extra seconds. For this particular exercise, this should be plenty for anyone to do.

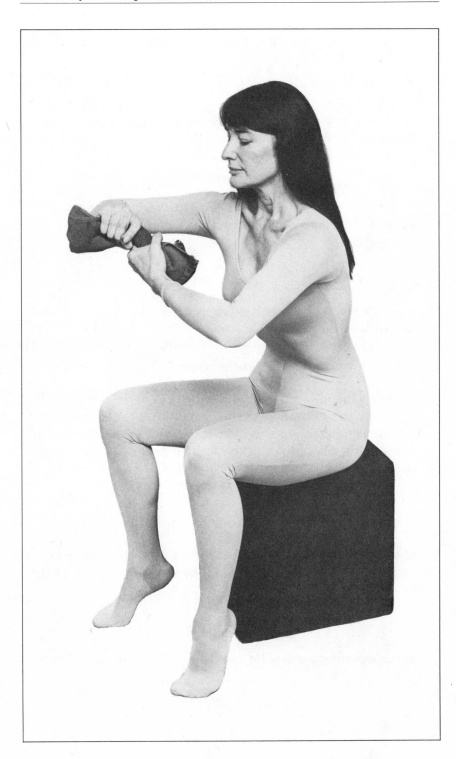

19. BACK-OF-ARM EXERCISE

What It Does

This gets the muscles of the backs of the upper arms smooth and tight.

Position

Sit down on a chair in front of a table or desk. Clear the surface and rest the whole forearm, from the elbow to the fist, on the surface.

Exercise

Tense the entire arm, press down into the table, and try to pull the arm slowly toward you.

Attention

(Use one hand for a moment to feel the back of the other arm to make sure the muscle down the back of the arm is tightened. You can also feel the large muscle at the back of your underarm by loosening the arm and then feeling the muscle tighten in your hand as you pull back with your arm.)

Try to put more effort into the exercise each day.

Caution

Before and after the following exercises do the flexibility exercise for the shoulders (page 57). Keep breathing throughout the exercise!

How Many

Do ten repetitions a day. Hold each time for six to ten seconds.

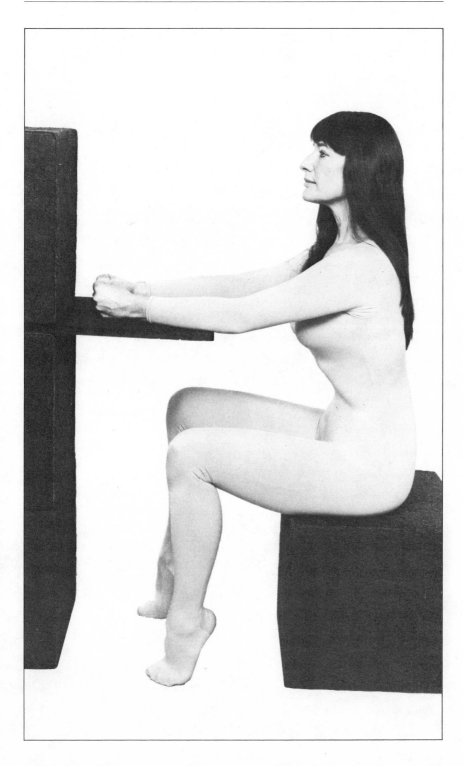

20. ALL-OVER STRETCH

What It Does

You can stretch your lower back, backs of your thighs, and the side muscles beautifully, all at the same time, with this exercise.

Caution

Use running in place (page 152) to warm up for these stretches.

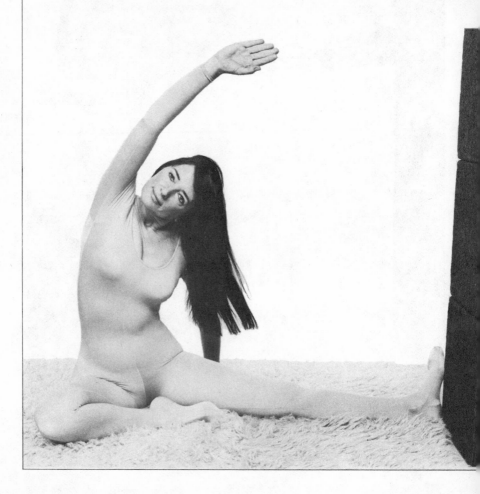

Position

Sit on the floor, facing a wall, with the left foot tucked in against the right thigh. Place the inside edge of the right foot against the wall. With your hands on the floor behind your back lean as far in toward the wall as possible. Try to make your back *feel* arched. Leave the right hand on the floor, elbow bent, to keep the back feeling arched. *Stretch the left arm straight up* from the shoulder in a line with your ear.

Exercise

Gently ease yourself into a stretch-out along the right leg. Try to keep your shoulders directly in line with that leg. Stretch as far down along the leg as possible. Bounce *gently* farther down along your leg. Keep your back straight always. Straighten the left elbow even more to get a better stretch.

When you are stronger, you can hold your back upright without the use of the arm braced on the floor. Lift both arms along your ears and stretch over to one side. Then stretch to the other side.

Attention

To stretch the inner thighs a little more each day before you begin or even during the exercise as you warm up, put both hands on the floor behind you and ease your bottom forward a little. You will feel your inner thigh stretch and tighten. Stretching takes time. Work gently and slowly. When you can, try this stretching exercise with both legs straight and with your feet against the wall.

How Many

Work up to eight or ten of these a day for each side.

Diet

15

Study
Your Own Body

Because we do much less physical labor than we did a hundred years ago, we need many fewer calories — but we still need to be very well nourished. *Those fewer calories must contain concentrated food value if we are to maintain our health!* The continued absence of necessary vitamins, minerals, and other components in extremely small amounts can cause us unnecessary disorders. Since we don't yet know all our nutritional needs, we ought to prefer the crude "natural" foods to the refined products of industry. For this reason a certain conservatism — being "old-fashioned" — seems the wisest approach.

There are also individual sensitivities and reactions that are not to be treated lightly. You must take the observations about your own body seriously and be alert for the ways in which you as an individual differ from others. These are the facts you must gather empirically — your personal experiences that serve to make you unique.

Among our individual differences are requirements for certain nutrients, vitamins, minerals, and the like. One person may need many times more or less of, say, a vitamin, than her neighbor does. There is no reliable minimum or maximum daily requirement. There are government studies that show individual differences to be so wide that any average is quite meaningless. You must, on the other hand, be aware of which vitamins and minerals are needed in certain amounts but can be toxic in other amounts.

If we ourselves are not completely knowledgeable about the whole combination of foods, we may leave out useful parts. Every year finds new and important nutrients discovered in the laboratories. Nobody pretends that biochemical or nutritional knowledge about foods — and in particular about subtle and rare trace components — is complete or even nearly complete. So it is extremely important to read labels and to opt for foods that have the fewest additives and have had no nutrients subtracted from them.

Every part of your body and its workings, with all the delicate timings and switches and seasonal changes, can break down for lack of the right food. It seems only sensible, when you have a disease or injury of any sort, when you have pain of any kind, when you have stress, when you have an emotional crisis to go through, when you have hard work to do, even if that work is only to continue existing, that one of the first things that should be attended to is diet, which is the source of repair. Even if your diet is good, there seems always to be room for improvement. This is a level on which you can positively help yourself. There is still a raft of diseases that are of unknown origin. A healthy body suffers disease less frequently and less severely than a body starved for one or another nutrient, whether or not one knows the cause of the disease. If the elements you are short of are not added, you cannot rebuild your body or even maintain its health, let alone improve it. If your body lets you know it needs something — by breaking out, hurting, getting too fat, too flabby or too thin, getting numb, getting overly fatigued or depressed — remember that you are the boss. Learn what to do about moving or feeding it better, and then do something about it!

As for getting fat, calories do *not* always count. Many women who have difficulty losing weight will eat less and less food, trying to lose their excess pounds. It seldom works. Without enough protein, the body holds fluids. Without enough potassium, the body holds fluids. With too much salt, the body holds fluids. Our hormonal balance also has a lot to do with our being overweight, as we see, for instance, each month just before menstruation. With the right food, you can sometimes double your intake of calories and lose weight. There are women who carry anywhere from five to fifty pounds of excess fluids. Without these fluids, they would be more comfortable and certainly less "fat"-looking. Being overweight is *not* necessarily being overly fat. But with some types of overweight, we may want to take supplements for insurance rather than add excessive calories.

We may miss getting what we need from our food each day. Our bodies for one reason or another (pregnancy, sickness, disease, old age) may not be processing our food as well as it should or may need more of some nutrients in times of stress. You can't rely on medicine to cure a disease caused by lack of the right foods, though you may be able to cover up the symptoms for a while. Nobody minds you betting on your death through so-called life insurance. Yet it's much more satisfying to invest in your life. Vitamins and minerals are a cheap form of real life insurance.

Insurance in the form of extra vitamins and minerals can be added best by adding them fresh. Try fresh vegetable and fruit juices. You'll need a juicer. If you have an overweight problem, stick with whole foods. As your body handles roughage, it burns calories.

If whole foods or juices add too many calories, use natural, organic vitamin supplements.

Take your vitamin-mineral tablets with a meal, never on an empty stomach.

The best food is almost good enough nowadays, but a little insurance never hurt anybody.

16

Protein

Every cell in the body is made up partly of protein, for all enzymes are protein, and so are a great many of the structured components. Our bodies use up protein every day, and when we do not get enough protein to replace what we have used, the body tissues do not get rebuilt to the proper specifications. Day by day you have a choice: rebuild or break down. Choose well. Every day's choice will show up ten years from now — if not next week.

Protein gives you the raw material; exercise does the building and developing. No animal, including man, survives without taking in protein.

To find out how much protein your body needs, decide what your proper weight *should* be, then divide that number by two. If you weigh 150 pounds and are normally active, you need about 75 grams of protein. This is generous. If you weigh 140, you need 70. If you are sick, injured, have a burn, or are under some other stress, you need more. Pregnant and nursing mothers may need half again as much protein.

As you get older, you do not digest proteins as well as you once did, so you may need to eat more protein-rich foods. At the end of this section, you'll find recipes for protein foods for people who have trouble chewing solid proteins.

Proteins are made of building blocks called amino acids. There are different amino acids that we need to build our tissues. Some can be converted into others by our body chemistry. Those that we can't make out of others we must take in. The proteins that we eat are broken down into their building blocks by digestion. But not all kinds of proteins have all the amino acids we need. These proteins are incomplete. Large amounts of incomplete proteins are usually found in carbohydrates, the higher calorie foods that we cannot afford to eat in quantity. It's easier just to make sure you're getting enough complete protein with *every meal.*

It is better to overdo on proteins than on any other food component. At the same time as everything is being rebuilt, some of the protein may be turned into carbohydrates and even from carbohydrates to fat. It is easier to lose fat, however, than to make up for lost protein.

Amount	Item	Protein (grams — approximate)	Calories (approximate)
¼ lb.	lean meat	20–30	215–280
¼ lb.	fish	20–30	150–200
¼ lb.	chicken, without skin	30–35	200–220
¼ lb.	shellfish	9–27	75–130
½ cup	cottage cheese	20	85–130
1 cup	soy flour (low fat)	37	313
8 oz.	yogurt (plain, low fat)	8.3	123
1 cup	wheat germ	80	440
1 tbsp.	yeast	8	80
1 cup	powdered milk	45	453

How much protein do *you* need a day?

How much did you have yesterday?

Write down everything you ate yesterday and then count the grams of protein.

Many people on weight-loss diets find they have to go off them because of weakness, faintness, even blacking out. This is usually caused by diets much too low in protein or potassium. A good diet has enough protein and potassium not only to prevent these problems but to make you feel much more cheerful and full of energy than you may normally feel.

If you work in the evenings or on a night shift, you need lots of protein at your evening meal. If you put in a working *day,* you should start it with protein. Always have protein before starting the *major work portion* of your day.

At your midwork break, instead of coffee, have some complete protein to keep your energy level high. A glass of milk or some cottage cheese, yogurt, or hard-boiled eggs will keep you feeling much better than coffee or coffee with pastries.

Have some complete protein with every meal to keep your body building itself. *And it needn't be expensive!* Soy flour, dried milk, yeast, and wheat germ give you the most for your money. You can add powdered milk to milk, custard, and gravies. Wheat germ can be used for breading or topping or as cereal or in baked goods. Yeast can be used in breads, pilafs, and stews. The uses of soy flour, soy grits, and soybeans are almost endless: baked beans, soups, soy nuts, soy pancakes, soy spoon bread, soy curd. Or try this:

Mix together: 1 cup soy flour
               1 cup wheat germ
               1 cup powdered milk
               ¼ cup yeast

This amounts to about fifty-five grams of protein per cup of mixture.

Store in the refrigerator in a tight container. Mix and use one cup — maybe less when you first start — in place of one cup of white flour in each recipe containing flour.

If your family likes snacks (and whose doesn't?), always have complete protein snacks around the house: cheese, soy nuts, milk, sardines, hard-boiled eggs, liver paste, yogurt, cottage cheese, canned shrimp, oysters, clams, lobster, and tuna (packed in water).

Since every cell in your body requires protein in order to stay healthy, be sure you get every gram of protein you need every day.

SOFT AND FAST PROTEIN RECIPES

These recipes will provide fast, high-protein foods for those with trouble chewing solid protein foods.

Egg Nogs

Mix: 1 cup milk (sweet acidophilus, if possible)
        1 to 3 tbsps. powdered milk
        1 or 2 eggs

Add: vanilla, or 1 teaspoon yeast and ½ banana, or 1 teaspoon yeast and a handful of almonds, or any nuts or seeds, or 1 teaspoon yeast and 1 tablespoon dark molasses or 1 tablespoon blackstrap molasses. (Start with a little blackstrap molasses; each of us is different.)

Cottage Cheese Salads

Add to cottage cheese any of the following: grated cheddar cheese, some lumps of blue cheese, a few tablespoons of applesauce, shrimp and curry powder, green onions and scissor-cut parsley, and crushed, unsweetened pineapple.

Fish Chowder #1

¼ pound any fish fillet, broken up in 1 cup of warm milk.

Mix 2 tablespoons of powdered milk with enough plain milk or water to make it smooth, and add it to the fish and milk. Keep it warm for a few minutes. Add herbs or spices as desired. Serve.

Fish Chowder #2 — Fillet Leftovers

Most fish markets will give you free fish leftovers from making fillets. Put skeleton, head and all, in pressure cooker. Cover with water and cook for 15 minutes at 15 pounds' pressure. Blend everything in blender. Fry onions and add to fish stock. Add as much milk, tomato juice, tomato-vegetable juice, or water as you like. Season as desired. Serve. Keep extra in freezer.

Blender Soups

Put 1 cup of hot milk into blender, start blender, and add 2 tablespoons of powdered milk.

Add one of these: small can of liver paste and ¼ teaspoon yeast
½ small can of lobster
½ small can of shrimp
½ small can of tuna
few spears of asparagus
big chunk of cheddar or other cheese
¼ cup of spinach
2 tablespoons of canned salmon

¼ peeled avocado
¼ cup of peas
Blend to desired consistency.

Desserts

To 1 cup of plain yogurt, add any one or mixture of the following:
  mashed banana
  applesauce (no sugar added)
  crushed pineapple (no sugar added)

Ice Cream

1 cup low-fat yogurt
6 generous tbsps. of frozen orange juice concentrate
¼ cup non-fat, non-instant powdered milk
1 banana
1 lemon wedge with skin
Put the yogurt, orange juice, and lemon in a blender. While blending, add the powdered milk and continue to blend for a few minutes. Then add the banana. Blend again to mix well. Poor into individual cups or a bowl. Cover with plastic wrap and freeze. For better flavor and texture, beat with an egg beater or electric mixer several times during freezing.

Snacks

canned liver pâté
canned sardines, in oil, water, mustard, or tomato sauce
canned salmon
seed cereal (see page 204), mixed in blender with milk or yogurt
If you can't drink milk, use fruit or fruit juice.

17
Potassium

It is obvious to almost all women that there is something going on with their bodies during the premenstrual period.

One of the major problems associated with the change in our diet from natural, unrefined foods to commercial, highly refined food products is caused by the shift in the amounts of sodium and potassium that we take in. Our bodies are built to reuse sodium — to hang on to it — but potassium is flushed through our systems relatively quickly.

Although both men and women are subject to the problems of our high-salt, low-potassium diets, in many women the effects are more pronounced and are apparent almost every month. Ten to twelve days before their menstrual periods, about 40 percent of all women dump potassium, losing it even faster than usual because of hormonal changes in the body. As a result, because potassium loss weakens muscles, many women feel weak, tired, and constipated, and even have nervous symptoms, because the brain is exceedingly sensitive to changes in the potassium-sodium balance.

When the sodium-potassium balance in the cells is changed, the excess sodium causes fluids to be held in the cells. Almost all of the other premenstrual symptoms can be related to this loss of potassium and consequent holding of fluids: vertigo, migraine, headaches, stuffy nose, hoarse voice, and tender breasts. When potassium is not replaced, many women suffer from this deficiency not just in the premenstrual days, but throughout the month. To date, there is no simple test, including a blood test, that will tell you what the potassium level is in your cells.

The only way to judge whether you have a potassium deficiency is by the symptoms. However, based on our modern diets, it is a fair assumption that few of us eat as much potassium as we need — and most of us eat far too much sodium. Once you know the situation, it isn't hard to correct this, but since the sodium-potassium balance is critical, it is just as important to decrease consumption of added sodium as it is to increase consumption of potassium. All you have to do is to eat natural, unprocessed foods and little salt. It is as simple a solution as it sounds.

The best sources of potassium are all naturally occurring foods — fish, fowl, fresh vegetables and fruits, whole grains, nuts, and meat. No food should be soaked unless the water is to be consumed, and if possible vegetables and fruits should be eaten raw. Sometimes the food products that are left over when foods are processed are those that are highest in potassium — for example, wheat germ, wheat bran, and blackstrap molasses. In many vegetables, the tops, which are commonly thrown away, are higher in potassium than the part of the vegetables we eat, such as turnip greens and beet tops.

There is no necessity for the average person to take potassium in a supplement, and no one should ever do so except on doctor's orders. Although the potassium chloride that is sold as a salt substitute is probably not harmful if taken only with food, potassium chloride in pill or liquid form is extremely irritating to the lining of the stomach and of the gut and can actually cause ulcerations.

On the other hand, there is no way that one can eat too much potassium in natural foods. Although excess salt is held on to by the body to a great extent, any excess potassium from food is simply harmlessly excreted.

CONSTIPATION

Women who suffer from chronic or premenstrual constipation should not take laxatives because they deplete the body of potassium. Lack of potassium slows down the workings of the colon and results in further constipation. It can also cause you to retain fluids. Taking diuretics can cause more potassium loss and more constipation.

A diet too low in fat can cause great difficulties in the easing of stool through the colon. An improperly low level of bulk or roughage constipates many people. So you need bulk to make the stool plump, oil to ease it through, potassium to keep normal action in the smooth muscles of the gut that grab the stool and push it along, and the right bacteria to help that internal compost heap, your stool.

Try this recipe instead of a laxative. Be sure to give it a couple of weeks' trial. Results are usually excellent.

Seed Cereal

Make a mixture of your favorite nuts and seeds. Use only the raw, unsalted variety. Any of the following are good:

sesame seeds	pecans
sunflower seeds	brazil nuts
pumpkin seeds	walnuts
	pignolas
	cashews
	hazel nuts

Make sure you have both nuts and seeds in the mixture; they work better together than alone. Add a few dried fruits, cut up, if you like. You may also add some wheat germ or bran or both. Added black-strap molasses gives more potassium and iron. If you don't like milk, serve the cereal over plain yogurt. With yogurt, this makes a meal, a snack, or a dessert.

18
Calcium and Magnesium

Just as it is impossible to discuss potassium without talking about sodium, calcium and magnesium must be considered together because they, too, must be present in the body in the proper proportion, which is about twice as much calcium as magnesium. The more calcium our diet contains, the more magnesium it must also have. Too little magnesium will result not only in a magnesium deficiency, but a loss of calcium, which will be excreted in the urine.

Thus, though we generally think of magnesium deficiencies in terms of symptoms of irritability and nervousness, too little magnesium can also be responsible for degenerative diseases of the teeth and bones. Because of this necessary balance between these two minerals, I have throughout this book recommended the use of dolomite, a compound in which calcium and magnesium are present in the correct balance, when a supplement is needed.

Although 99 percent of all the calcium in our bodies is in our bones and teeth, the remaining 1 percent, which circulates through the blood and supplies the soft tissues, is of vital importance in the functioning of nerves and muscles, the regulation of the heartbeat, and the clotting of blood. Mild deficiencies of this tiny amount of blood calcium can lead to menstrual cramps, muscle cramps in the legs or feet, backaches, nervousness, irritability, and tremors.

CALCIUM

In women, the amount of calcium in the blood drops sharply a week or two prior to menstruation and is, partially at least, the cause of premenstrual tension and anxiety attacks. At the time of actual menstruation, the blood calcium drops further and can cause menstrual cramps.

Many women suffer from rather severe calcium deficiency starting around the age of forty and continuing from then on. There is a slowdown and finally a cessation of hormone production from the ovaries, which causes a sharp drop in blood calcium. Backaches, hot flashes, irritability, and depression are linked to this calcium loss.

As women age, the most serious result of calcium deficiency is osteoporosis (literally, porous bones). This often causes backs to ache and hips and forearms to break. It may be related to a lack of calcium in the diet or to a Vitamin D^3 deficiency or both. Unless Vitamin D^3 is present in adequate amounts, the body is unable to absorb calcium from food. The body manufactures its own Vitamin D^3 in the presence of sunshine. The only good food source of this Vitamin D^3 is cod liver oil. If you cannot take cod liver oil in oil form daily, take cod liver oil capsules.

The best food sources of calcium are milk and milk products, including cheese and yogurt. Eat these foods with fruit or vegetables to maintain a calcium-magnesium balance.

		Calcium
skim milk	8 oz.	296 mgs.
whole milk	8 oz.	288 mgs.
yogurt	8 oz.	264 mgs.
Parmesan cheese	1 oz.	383 mgs.
cheddar cheese	1 oz.	213 mgs.
blue cheese	1 oz.	207 mgs.
Swiss cheese	1 oz.	160 mgs.

If you cannot digest milk, here are a few inexpensive ways to get calcium:

Eggshell soup stock: Save your eggshells, put them in the blender with a little water, and pulverize them. Put the mixture in a pot with about 1 pint of water and either a tomato or 1 tablespoon of wine or vinegar. Simmer for an hour. Strain and add more water to make about 1 pint of stock. Use the stock for a soup base.

Beef-bone soup stock: Cover beef bones with water, add a tomato or wine or vinegar (the acid in these helps dissolve the calcium from the bones), and cook slowly for several hours. You can also make this stock in a pressure cooker. To all of the above, add many vegetables or beans for their magnesium content.

MAGNESIUM

Seventy percent of the magnesium in the body is contained in the bones and teeth; the rest is an essential component of all the soft tissues. It is vital for nerve and muscle function. Use of alcohol seriously depletes the body's magnesium supply. Since our usual daily intake of magnesium is low, drinking cocktails as a regular habit can give you serious problems.

We are getting considerably less magnesium in our foods today than our grandparents did. In 1910, the average magnesium intake per person each day was 408 milligrams. Today's average is a little over 100 milligrams. The main reason for this decrease is that we eat less bread and cereal than our ancestors did — and the bread and cereal that we do eat has been refined. Whole wheat flour has more than four times as much magnesium as "enriched" white flour. In spite of the food manufacturers' claims about enrichment and fortification, not everything that has been removed from food in processing and refining is returned. Magnesium is one of the nutrients that is not replaced.

Another cause of the decline of magnesium in our diets is the increased use of chemical fertilizers. Chemical fertilizers inhibit the absorption of magnesium by plants from the soil. This is a good reason to grow your own vegetables or to buy organically grown foods.

The best food sources of magnesium are whole grains and dried beans, peas, and nuts. Soybeans and peanuts are excellent sources. Fresh, raw, green leafy vegetables are also excellent magnesium suppliers.

WHAT YOU CAN DO

Monthly or constant nervousness and irritability are signs of a magnesium and calcium deficiency. A teaspoon of dolomite powder mixed in orange juice or cider and taken with cod liver oil is a marvelous calmative, excellent to use in cases of hyperventilation, anxiety attacks, insomnia, tension, or nervousness. After the age of forty, all women probably should take this mixture nightly before bed and at other times as seems necessary to calm nerves and anxieties. (Cod liver oil is needed just once a day.)

Since the body can absorb calcium only at a steady rate, calcium is lost during any period of fasting. Calcium must be supplied steadily, especially just before sleeping and at breakfast. Most calcium is lost during sleep from the combination of a long fasting period between dinner and breakfast and the lack of the pull of muscle when you are lying relaxed. This is another reason why we must not sit a lot during the day. Weight on the bones, the pull of the muscle against the bone, helps us to conserve our calcium.

When your body is under stress, you can lose more calcium than you take in. You may need to repeat the amount of dolomite you take. Your body will say it needs it by producing cramps or anxiety. Where digestion may be poor, or when fast action is desired, the powder form of dolomite works best because it is already broken up to some extent. Calcium will deposit in soft tissues, kidneys, and arteries only if it is not supplied to the body with magnesium. That is why dolomite, with the proper two-to-one balance, is the preferred supplement.

A more popular supplement, though not quite as good as dolomite, is a glass of hot milk with one tablespoon of blackstrap molasses. The molasses gives you magnesium and iron along with the calcium. Make sure you also have calcium with each meal or with snacks.

Your doctor should be discussing these conditions with you as you deal with them. Any more serious problems with your calcium-magnesium balance will need his or her experienced eye.

19

Fertilizer for Humans

Some very high-quality foods eaten every day can give you all the elements and compounds we know, so far, that you need, plus some other components yet to be discovered or separated out. That sentence is the key! We do not know yet all those things that are necessary for optimal health. To assure ourselves of a much better diet, a little "fertilizer" is in order.

In the following recipe, all your daily needs seem well accounted for in the light of most commonly agreed-on nutritional requirements. All that is said to be required is in there, as well as more of certain nutrients that have been found to be necessary. The concoction is awful in taste but small in amount, is low in calories, and is a highly sustaining base for weight reduction.

All new foods take getting used to. Start slowly with 1 teaspoon of the dry ingredients and ½ teaspoon of the oils added to 8 ounces of water, juice, or milk. (Milk will give you 7 additional grams of protein.) Start a blender with the liquid in it and add the dry ingredients and the oils. If you don't have a blender, shake the mixture in the above order in a jar. Increase amounts daily over two or three weeks until you are using a heaping ¼ cup of dry ingredients and 1 tablespoon plus 1 teaspoon of the mixed oils each time.

This is what goes into The Brew daily, if you take a heaping ¼ cup of dry ingredients plus 1 tablespoon and 1 teaspoon of the oils:

Powders: 3 heaping tbsps. yeast
1 heaping tbsp. desiccated liver
1 tsp. each: bone meal
dolomite
lecithin, granulated
¼ tsp. kelp
Oils: 1 tsp. high-potency cod liver oil
1 tsp. soy oil
2 tsps. wheat germ oil
Add: 1 acidophilus capsule (emptied into The Brew daily)
½ tsp. Vitamin C granules
1 tbsp. molasses (Grandma's Dark)

These products may be bought in a health-food store or by mail order.

(A brand name has been given in one case only because I find its quality and flavor attractive.)

Some people may be allergic to torula yeast; they should use brewer's yeast. If oils "repeat," try taking up the level more slowly or taking the oils with a meal or before going to bed. (In this case take the dry ingredients mixed with water or juice in the morning.) If you find dried liver distasteful, eat ⅛ pound of cooked liver daily at any meal.

I can't promise that The Brew's flavor is easy to get used to. Try holding your breath, using a straw, gulping it down . . . I've tried to make substitutions, but have never found as good a balance of ingredients that tastes any better. The Brew gives you all the suggested day's needs in vitamins, minerals, and most of your protein. Whatever the cost (about $.50 a day), it is an excellent food bargain, because you get everything needed in known nutrients for a full day, in everything but calories and roughage — all of that, in just "one moment of madness"!!

The Brew contains 395 calories.

Ten-Day
Diet for Women

You are unique! No one else — *ever* — in the world will be quite like you. Never seriously look for yourself on charts; charts can give you only a vague idea, not exact information. To know what you really should weigh, look at yourself stripped in front of a mirror — profile and back, too! When, with a combination of dieting and exercise, you look good to *yourself,* that is what you should weigh. Never think of yourself as an "average."

You cannot diet away flabby muscles. You cannot do the whole job with diet, just as you cannot do the whole job with exercise. You must exercise too! *The exercise is as important as the food!*

Everyone should know how to count calories. In a world full of machines to do our work, and of processed foods to fool our bodies, it is much more important to count calories and know what vitamins and minerals there are in food than it is to be a gourmet cook or a beautiful table-setter — though these qualities are quite nice to have.

People in good health who are ten pounds or more overweight can safely lose ten pounds in ten days. If you have any doubt about your health, *ask your doctor.*

The one thing that wrecks weight-loss diets faster than anything else is cheating. And the one thing that creates cheaters faster than anything else is a diet that doesn't satisfy in texture, color, or quantity, or one that is much too complicated. This diet is for ten days, giving you the same foods for each of those ten days; so simple and so satisfying (and so boring), it is easy to follow and succeed with.

The reason most crash diets are seven to ten days long is that by the end of this period your body readjusts. Much excess body water has been lost. After this point is reached, taking off the excess fat is a longer, slower process.

In this diet, there is plenty of protein in the milk, yogurt, wheat germ, sardines, tuna, and liver to keep up your energy level. There are plenty of needed vitamins and minerals in all the foods, including the very important potassium, calcium, and iron, to keep you healthy. There is plenty of roughage to keep you from getting constipated. In other words, food value is high, calories are low. The only rule — the *unbreakable rule* — is: no additions, no subtractions, no substitutions, except as noted.

THE TEN-DAY DIET

Breakfast:	1 tbsp. bran	31 *Calories*
	1 tbsp. wheat germ	24
	1 tbsp. blackstrap molasses	43
	1 cup skim milk (or low-fat yogurt)	89 (123)
		187 (221)
Lunch:	4 oz. unsalted sardines, drained (or canned pink salmon)	200 *Calories*
	6 leaves loose-leaf lettuce	15
	1 tsp. oil	32
	1 tsp. lemon juice	4
		251
Dinner:	1 cup mushrooms	41 *Calories*
	¼ lb. liver	250
	6 leaves loose-leaf lettuce	15
	1 cup parsley	25
	1 tsp. sweet butter	25
		306
Late-Night Snack:	1 cup skim milk or yogurt	89 *Calories*
	1 tbsp. blackstrap molasses	43
	1 tsp. cod liver oil	35
		167
	Plus 8 cups of water with lemon	24 *Calories*
Total		935 Calories

Use as little salt as possible. The use of any spices and herbs to make the diet more interesting is perfectly acceptable — in flavoring amounts only.

Have liver at least two or three times a week. On the other days, choose other proteins: chicken (no skin)

> clams
> shrimp
> lobster
> sweetbreads

BEST FOODS IN ALL CATEGORIES

These foods are low in calories, much higher in potassium than sodium, and well balanced in calcium and magnesium. The foods included are also high in other minerals and in vitamins. If processing is involved, it is to concentrate vitamins, minerals, protein, bacteria, and roughage to give you more food value in fewer calories.

Nuts, grains, seeds (raw)

rice bran	brazil nuts	(Although these are
wheat bran	hazel nuts	high in calories, the
wheat germ	peanuts	sodium, potassium,
sunflower seeds	coconut (unsweetened)	and magnesium
pumpkin seeds	pecans	content are so
soybeans	pistachios	concentrated that you
almonds		should include at least
sesame seeds		a few in your daily
		diet.)

Vegetables

Brussels sprouts	parsley	(* Take more of these
cauliflower	broccoli	foods during the two
chicory	*beet greens	premenstrual weeks.)
endive	mushrooms	
kale	turnips	
spinach	sweet potato (with	
parsnips	skin)	
watercress	white potato (with	
*turnip greens	skin)	
	*collards	

Dairy (all dairy products should be low fat)

yogurt
buttermilk
milk
kephir
cultured cottage cheese (unsalted, uncreamed)

(Be sure to take fruits or vegetables with milk products to bring up the potassium-magnesium balance.)

Meats (lean, broiled, or sautéed at medium heat with little or no fat)

kidney
beef liver
calf liver
veal
flank steak
hamburger

(All meat, fowl, and fish are low in calcium, except for sardines and salmon.)

Fowl

giblets
chicken

turkey
duck

Fish

flounder
haddock
halibut
snapper
cod
herring
salmon (no salt)

mussels
sardines (no salt)
crab
clams
lobster
shrimp

(If you still gain some weight or fluid in the premenstrual period, take fewer of these foods in your diet.)

Seaweeds

dulse
Irish moss
kelp

(See comment above.)

Other excellent sources of nutrients

*dark molasses
brewer's yeast
torula yeast
"Super" yeast

(* Take more in the two premenstrual weeks.)

Whole grains and legumes

whole wheat   (These are good sources but higher in
whole rye   carbohydrates. If you have no weight problem, use
whole cornmeal   them.)
brown rice
split peas
barley
oats

Fruits

apricots
avocados
cantaloupe
mangoes
peaches
plantains
prunes

Doctors and Medications

21
Visiting the Doctor

Too often the symptoms that sent us to the doctor seem to disappear in a cloud of confusion when we are finally in the office. You can help your doctor to help you if you write down all the symptoms as you think of them *before* your visit. Take enough time to write all the information completely and clearly so that nothing is missed.

What part of you is in trouble?
Where?
When did it start this time?
Has it ever happened before?
When does it happen?
How often?
More often now than before?
Mostly when you're in one position?
Which position?
Does the part look or feel different to you?
How?
What kind of discomfort do you have?
How long does it last?
Does anything else tend to happen at the same time?
How long does it last?
How does it affect you?
What have you been doing for it?
For how long?
Does it come on suddenly?
What were you doing just before it happened?
Has any member of your family had such a problem?

In addition, write down the answers to the following questions. If your doctor doesn't ask you these questions, be sure to give him or her the information yourself.

Do you have any allergies to food or drugs?
Are you taking any other drugs now?
Which ones?
What for?
Are you pregnant?
Are you breast-feeding?

If the doctor you are seeing is not your regular doctor, arrange to have your medical records sent to the new doctor. You may want to ask the secretary to get your medical records for you.

Any time spent in a doctor's office is a time of stress. Few people under stress remember all they've been told by the doctor. So as not to make mistakes, get your doctor or the secretary to help you understand the directions and to follow them better by *writing down* for you

- the possible diagnosis
- what he or she wants you to do at home or work, and how often
- what tests he or she wants you to have taken
- what medication he or she wants you to take, how often, and how long
- generic name of the medication (cheaper though usually of the same quality)
- possible side effects to watch for
- any foods to avoid while taking this prescription
- any other drugs to avoid
- whether you should take the medication with food or on an empty stomach
- whether you should get up at night to take the medication
- whether you should stop taking the medication when you feel better or till it's used up, or whether you should refill the prescription
- how often she or he wants to hear from you
- when she or he wants you to return (day, hour, place)

22
Buying and Taking Medications

Ask your doctor or pharmacist to label the medication as to what it is being given for.

Always get from your pharmacist the enclosure that accompanies the medication, and read the enclosure at least twice to learn about all the possible side effects. On the unlikely chance that you do have any problems caused by the drug, you can then possibly recognize them. There *is* a need to know what could happen so that you can deal with your body intelligently.

After you have received the medication, ask the druggist to repeat exactly what the medication is and how it is to be taken. Many pharmacists give this information without being asked and will repeat it if you ask.

Be cautious! Women seem to react more strongly to drugs and to have more adverse side effects to them than men do.

Older people, more often than younger ones, may react abnormally to medication. If you are older, try to take your first one or two doses of a new medication when there are other people around.

When pregnant or nursing, do not take any drugs unless your doctor feels they are absolutely necessary. You want to avoid any possible harm to the fetus or baby, of course.

Mark on the bottle or box every time you take your medication so that you won't make mistakes in dosage. Medicine containers should have a time chart on the side to make this easy for you. You can always make a chart and tape it to the side of the containers.

No. of pills   Time   How many to take   How many left

People who are on sedatives or under stress or those who are simply forgetful often lose track of when they last took medication. You can see the danger in this.

You must never take more medication than has been specified by your doctor. Serious side effects can occur with some medications even at a normal dosage. Many drugs are very strong in their action, so don't double up on medication if you missed a dose. Instead, set your alarm clock in time for the next dose, unless you are instructed otherwise. Reread instructions to be sure you're taking the dosages properly. If you do have side effects of any sort (dizziness, faintness, depressions, fatigue, rashes — anything that happens that has not happened before), *stop the medication and call your doctor!* If you know (and you should know), tell the doctor what medication you are taking. Be ready to describe how the medication looks (color, size, shape, indentations, initials) and the dosage. There's always the remote chance you've been given the wrong medication or the wrong dosage. This information can help your doctor decide. If the effects are serious, call a friend or neighbor first or let the phone operator know where you are! Give her your phone number. Then call your doctor no matter what the time. If you can't reach your doctor, try another doctor or get yourself to a hospital emergency room. In any case:

- Be sure to store drugs as directed (refrigerate, keep dry, and so on).
- Do not take other people's medications.
- Do not offer other people your medication.
- Do not mix drugs except on your doctor's advice.
- Do not transfer medication from the original container without consulting your pharmacist.
- Check to find out whether alcoholic beverages are compatible with your medication, if you drink.
- Don't take drugs that are not dated recently.
- Recheck the label each time before taking medication.
- Throw away all old drugs.
- Keep all medications concealed and out of the reach of children.

- Never take medication for longer than the prescribed time without rechecking with your doctor to see whether she or he wishes you to continue.
- But do not stop taking the medication without consulting your doctor. Work *with* your doctor or find another one you can work with.

23

Operations and Serious Illness

There comes a time in most people's lives when a serious physical problem will arise. Strong medications may be needed, operations suggested, or serious tests proposed.

What is the right thing to do? Many women will have a family doctor or a few specialists with whom they have always dealt. This is the common-sense way to handle most problems. More serious troubles, however, require a different strategy: *you need to get a second opinion*

- because almost every medication has its side effects.
- because every time you have surgery there are related problems to be faced, for example, with the anesthesia.
- because tests may also have serious side effects and possible complications.
- because the most dedicated and intelligent and learned doctor does not know everything.

This is your body. Treat it with great respect. Get all possible information pro and con before making any decisions.

In the early stages it is best if the doctors that you consult for opinions are not closely connected to each other. This ensures that you will get possible differences of opinion on the medical problem. Then get your doctors to work together. That does not mean that you do not question them. You must understand them. You must know the reasons for the decisions that are going to affect your life.

Good doctors, in every case I have come across, enjoy discussing an interesting case with a colleague. Be wary of doctors who are irritated with your wanting a second opinion. In your place they would insist on one — or two! Many, in fact, make intensive studies before anyone lays a hand on them for surgery.

You think you can't afford another doctor? A second opinion? What you really cannot afford is unnecessary surgery or a permanent, and perhaps irremediable, change in your body that does not leave you better off. Ask these questions of each doctor you see and write down the answers or have the doctor write down the answers:

What do you (the doctor) feel is the probable diagnosis?
What do you feel should be done?
When?
By whom?
How long will I be laid up?
How much improvement can I expect?
What are the possible problems that can ensue during
     treatment?
After treatment?
Will there have to be any long-term or expensive follow-up
     treatment?
What are each of the tests for? What are the possible side
     effects?
How much will it cost? How much time will it take me
     away from home or family or work?
If drugs are a part of the treatment, what are the possible
     side effects?
What are the long-term effects to be had from medication?
     Surgery? Other suggested treatment?
Does this shorten my life span?
What things will it prevent me from doing that I can do now?
How long will that be the case?
What chance is there that there will be problems if I
     decide against the treatment suggested?
What alternatives do I have?

Armed with this information, settle yourself down to think about what your decision would be if this were not about yourself. Difficult? Yes. But necessary if you are going to bring good judgment to bear on your problem.

Try not to be rushed into making a decision. Of course, this is not always possible in case of accident or emergency. Even under such circumstances, if there's time, get a second opinion.

HAVING YOUR OVARIES REMOVED

For clarity's sake, we will define the terms used for removal of the ovaries and the uterus. Hysterectomy is removal of the uterus. Oophorectomy is removal of one or both ovaries. Oophorohysterectomy is removal of the ovaries and the uterus.

Having your ovaries removed *does* change you — permanently. Ovaries continue to function after removal of the uterus until the patient reaches the normal age of menopause (whenever that may be) and even afterward in a reduced capacity. Retaining your ovaries seems to protect you against coronary artery disease and osteoporosis.

There are almost three times the number of strokes in women who have had their ovaries removed as in those who have retained them. Removal of ovaries catapults you into instant and early menopause, with all its changes. These rapid and drastic hormonal changes are physically and emotionally draining. You will tend to have higher serum cholesterol after your ovaries are removed.

According to Dr. T. L. T. Lewis, of Queen Charlotte's Hospital for Women, in England, who reported his findings at the 1975 Symposium on Menopause and the Postmenopausal Years, the incidence of malignancy in ovaries is very low: 0.3 to 2 percent (from three to twenty women in a thousand). Depression is four times as common, more severe, and longer, following removal of ovaries, than with any other major surgery. Get a second opinion before having surgery. Hang on to your ovaries unless they are clearly diseased. Of course, in case of proven malignancy, the ovaries must be removed.

After either partial or complete hysterectomies — whether removal of the uterus alone or of the uterus and ovaries — some women have continued weight problems. Hormonal therapy, dangerous in itself, doesn't necessarily prevent weight problems.

BREAST CANCER

When measured in terms of survival of the patient, radical mastectomies are no better than simple mastectomies. Nevertheless, radical mastectomies continue to be a favored mode of treatment, even though experimental trials have shown that for most cases of breast cancer characterized as local, radical mastectomy is no more effective for long-term survival than the far less mutilating procedure, lumpectomy plus radiation.

This information comes from the following papers. The papers and the authors' references are available to every concerned woman through most local library search services.

Fox, Maurice S., Ph.D., "On the Diagnosis and Treatment of Breast Cancer," *The Journal of the American Medical Association,* February 2, 1979, vol. 241.

Bailar, John C., III, M.D., "A Time for Caution," Presented at the International Symposium on the Late Biological Effects on Ionizing Radiation, Vienna, March 15, 1978.

PLASTIC SURGERY

The worst problem with plastic surgery is that it's too damned expensive! Where it is needed, it should be provided. Even if some cases for which it is needed are not life-threatening, it certainly can be "quality of life"–threatening. Imagine yourself with one of these problems:

1. Breasts that continue to grow and grow, becoming larger, heavier, more pendulous year by year.
2. You have carried twins or more or have carried much fluid with a pregnancy or have lost a lot of weight so that a large flap of abdominal skin hangs in a fold reaching down over your thighs.
3. You have had an abdominal operation, and the resulting scar looks as if a seamstress had put in gathers or pleats.
4. You have had a breast removed, and don't see any reason why you should resign yourself to the way you look.

Would you deny yourself plastic surgery in any of these cases? Each of these cases is not just uncomfortable; it may be grotesque.

It also costs more to buy outsize or different clothing. Living, in many of these cases, is changed drastically because where you go and what you can do is cut down by how easily you can move and what you can wear.

Wouldn't it be nice if all necessary surgery were performed with two surgeons? One to pluck out or repair what offends you, and the other a plastic surgeon so that you needn't be reminded of the operation every day of your life? If we smash up a car, we return it as much as possible to its former state if we care about our investment. Why not our own bodies?

Short-term disasters to our bodies, such as burns or accidents, are acceptable in our eyes as good reasons for plastic surgery. Why not long-term disasters? And among those is aging, or a feature we can't stand. Where is the great virtue in letting your life happen to you, with you exerting no control? Plastic surgery for looking good is called optional, which means that psychological harm is not counted as impairment of function. If you used the same standard in your daily life, you would not repair your house, carry insurance, have bank accounts. And who decides what is a disaster? A doctor? Your friends? You live *your* life in *your* body. *You* get to choose! But, sad to say, only if you've got enough money, at least when it comes to plastic surgery.

If you're going to have work done, be sure to get the best plastic surgeon you can afford.

Bibliography

Bibliography

BOOKS

Alexander, Stewart F., M.D.; D. Farage; W. E. Hassan, Jr.; and R. D. Martin (assoc. ed.). *Hazards of Medication: A Manual on Drug Interactions, Incompatibilities, Contraindications, and Adverse Effects.* Philadelphia and Toronto: J. B. Lippincott Co., 1971.

Barnes, Cyril G. *Medical Disorders in Obstetric Practice* (4th ed.). Oxford, London, Edinburgh, Melbourne: Blackwell Scientific Publications, 1974.

Basmajian, J. V., M.D. *Grant's Method of Anatomy.* Baltimore: Williams and Wilkins Co., 1971.

Beard, R. J. *The Menopause: A Guide to Current Research and Practice.* Baltimore: University Park Press, 1976.

Becker, Frederick R.; James W. Wilson; and John A. Gehweiler. *The Anatomical Basis of Medical Practice.* Baltimore: Williams and Wilkins Co., 1971.

Berenberg, S. R., M.D. *Puberty, Biologic and Psychosocial Components.* Leiden: H. D. Stenfert Kroese B.V., 1975.

Campbell, Stuart. *The Management of the Menopause and Post-Menopausal Years.* Baltimore: University Park Press, 1976.

Carlson, Lars A., M.D. *Nutrition in Old Age: Symposia of the Swedish Nutrition Foundation.* Stockholm: Almqvist and Wiksell, 1972.

Church, Charles F.; and Helen N. Church. *Food Values of Portions Commonly Used* (12th ed.). Philadelphia: J. B. Lippincott Co., 1975.

Dalton, Katharina, MRCS, LRCP. *The Premenstrual Syndrome.* Springfield, Illinois: Charles C. Thomas, Publisher, 1964.

Damon, Albert; Howard W. Stoudt; and Ross A. McFarland. *The Human Body in Equipment Design.* Cambridge: Harvard University Press, 1971.

Donovan, B. T., Ph.D.; and J. D. VanDerWerff Ten Bosch, M.D. *Physiology of Puberty.* Baltimore: Williams and Wilkins Co., 1965.

Fox, H.; and F. A. Langley. *Postgraduate Obstetrical and Gynæcological Pathology.* Oxford: Pergamon Press, 1973.

Frisch, Rose E. "Food Intake, Fatness, and Reproductive Ability." In *Anorexia Nervosa,* R. A. Vigersky, ed. New York: Raven Press, 1977.

Hawkins, D. F., D.Sc. *Obstetric Therapeutics, Clinical Pharmacology, and Therapeutics in Obstetric Practice.* Baltimore: Williams and Wilkins Co., 1974.

Hoppenfeld, Stanley, M.D. *Physical Examination of the Spine and Extremities.* New York: Appleton-Century-Crofts, 1976.

Hytten, Frank E.; and Isabella Leitch. *The Physiology of Human Pregnancy.* Oxford: Blackwell Scientific Publications, 1964.

Kapandji, I. A. *The Physiology of the Joints:* vol. 1, *The Upper Limb;* vol. 2, *The Lower Limb;* and vol. 3, *The Trunk and the Vertebral Column.* Edinburgh, London, and New York: Churchill Livingstone, 1974.

Kaplan, Helen Singer, M.D. *The New Sex Therapy: Active Treatment of Sexual Dysfunctions.* New York: Brunner/Mazel Publishers, 1974.

Katchadourian, Herant A., M.D.; and D. T. Lunde, M.D. *Fundamentals of Human Sexuality* (2nd ed.). New York, London, Sydney: Stanford University, Holt, Rinehart, and Winston, 1975.

Krusen, Frank H., M.D.; Frederic J. Kottke, M.D.; and Paul M. Ellwood, M.D. *Handbook of Physical Medicine and Rehabilitation.* Philadelphia, London, Toronto: W. B. Saunders Co., 1971.

Licht, Sidney, M.D. *Rehabilitation and Medicine.* Baltimore: Waverly Press, Inc., 1968.

———. *Therapeutic Exercise* (2nd ed. rev.). Baltimore: Waverly Press, Inc., 1965.

Masters, William H., and Virginia E. Johnson. *Human Sexual Inadequacy.* Boston: Little, Brown and Co., 1970.

Michele, Arthur A., M.D. *Iliopsoas, Development of Anomalies in Man.* Springfield, Illinois: Charles C. Thomas, Publisher, 1962.

Mountcastle, Vernon B. *Medical Physiology,* 2 vols. (13th ed.) Saint Louis: The C. V. Mosby Co., 1974.

Myles, Margaret F., S.R.N.; H. V. Cert; and Sister Tutor Cert, M.T. *Textbook for Midwives with Modern Concepts of Obstetric and Neonatal Care.* Edinburgh, London, and New York: Churchill Livingstone, 1975.

Romney, Seymour L., M.D.; M. J. Gray; A. B. Little; J. A. Merrill; E. J. Quilligan; and R. Stander. *Gynecology and Obstetrics: The Health Care of Women.* New York: McGraw-Hill Book Co., A Blakiston Publication, 1975.

Ruch, Theodore C., Ph.D; and Harry D. Patton, Ph.D., M.D. *Physiology and Biophysics* (19th ed.). Philadelphia and London: W. B. Saunders Co., 1966.

Van Cott, Harold P., Ph.D; and Robert G. Kinkade, Ph.D. *Human Engineering Guide to Equipment Design* (rev. ed.). Washington, D.C.: American Institutes for Research, 1972.

Warwick, Roger; and Peter L. Williams. *Gray's Anatomy* (35th British ed.). Philadelphia: W. B. Saunders Co., 1973.

Watt, Bernice K.; and A. L. Merrill. *Composition of Foods, Raw, Processed,*

Prepared. Agricultural Handbook No. 8 (rev. ed.). Washington, D.C.: U.S. Department of Agriculture, Agricultural Research Service, December 1963.

PERIODICALS

Applegate, W. V.; Alan Forsythe; and J. B. Bauernfeind. "Physiological and Psychological Effects of Vitamin E and B6 on Women Taking Oral Contraceptives." *International Journal of Vitamins and Nutrition Research,* 49 (1979).

Ayres, S., Jr.; and R. Mihan. "Nocturnal Leg Cramps (Systremma) — A Progress Report on Response to Vitamin E." *Southern Medical Journal,* 67 (November 1974), no. 11.

Backstrom, T.; and B. Mattson. "Correlation of Symptoms in Premenstrual Tension to Oestrogen and Progesterone Concentrations in Blood Plasma." *Neuropsychobiology,* 1 (1975).

Backstrom, Torbjorn; H. Carstensen; R. Sodergard; and L. Wide. "FSH, LH, TeBg-Capacity. Estrogen and Progesterone in Women with Premenstrual Tension During the Luteal Phase." *Journal of Steroid Biochemistry,* 7 (1976).

Bailor, John D., III, M.D. "A Time for Caution." *Breast Disease.* Proceedings of International Symposium, May 13–17, 1978. New York: Grune and Stratton Rapid Manuscript Reproduction, 1978.

Bayliss, R. I. S.; and O. M. Edwards. "Idiopathic Oedema of Women: A Clinical and Investigative Study." *Quarterly Journal of Medicine,* New Series, 45 (January 1976), no. 177.

Bell, B.; M. J. Christie; and P. H. Venables. "Menstrual Cycle Variation in Body Fluid Potassium." *Journal of Interdisciplinary Cycle Research,* 6 (1975), no. 2.

Berens, Stephen C.; J. M. Davis; and D. S. Janowsky. "Correlations Between Mood, Weight, and Electrolytes During the Menstrual Cycle: A Renin-Angiotensin-Aldosterone Hypothesis of Premenstrual Tension." *Psychosomatic Medicine,* 35 (March–April 1973), no. 2.

Beshear, Donna R.; K. T. Roberts; and W. D. Snively. "The Sodium-Restricted Diet Revised." *The Journal of the Indiana State Medical Association,* 67 (December 1974), no. 12.

Brush, M. G. "The Possible Mechanisms Causing the Premenstrual Tension Syndrome." *Current Medical Research and Opinion,* 4 (1977), suppl. 4.

Clare, A. W. "Psychological Profiles of Women Complaining of Premenstrual Symptoms." *Current Medical Research and Opinion,* 4 (1977), suppl. 4.

Dalton, Katharina. "Premenstrual Syndrome." *Update,* July 1975.

Daly, Veronica; G. Herrman; S. Hineman; and M. Schuckit. "Premenstrual Symptoms and Depression in a University Population." *Diseases of the Nervous System,* September 1975.

DeLuca, Hector F. "Function of Fat-Soluble Vitamins." *The American Journal of Clinical Nutrition*, 28 (April 1975).

Department of Health, Education, and Welfare. "Health Effects of the Pregnancy Use of Diethylstilbestrol." *Physician Advisory*, October 4, 1978.

———. "Update on Estrogens and Uterine Cancer." *Food and Drug Administration Drug Bulletin*, 9 (February–March 1979), 1.

———. "We Want You to Know About Prescription Drugs" (pamphlet, HEW Publication No. [FDA] 78-3059). Rockville, Maryland: Public Health Service, Food and Drug Administration, Office of Public Affairs.

Doig, A.; E. A. Michie; and J. Parboosingh. "Changes in Renal Water and Electrolyte Excretion Occurring Before and After Induced Ovulation and Their Relation to Total Oestrogen and Pregnanediol Excretion." *The Journal of Obstetrics and Gynæcology of the British Commonwealth*, New Series, 81 (June 1974), no. 6.

Farrell, P. M.; and J. G. Bieri. "Megavitamin E Supplementation in Man." *American Journal of Clinical Nutrition*, 28 (1975), no. 12.

Field, Peggy Anne; and J. Funke. "The Premenstrual Syndrome: Current Findings, Treatment, and Implications for Nurses." *JOGN Nursing*, September–October 1976.

Fox, Maurice S. "On the Diagnosis and Treatment of Breast Cancer." *Journal of the American Medical Association*, 241 (February 2, 1979), no. 5.

Frisch, Rose E. "Population, Food Intake, and Fertility." *Science*, 199 (January 6, 1978).

———; and J. W. McArthur. "Menstrual Cycles: Fatness as a Determinant of Minimum Weight for Height Necessary for Their Maintenance or Onset." *Science*, 185 (September 13, 1974).

Garvin, James E.; T. W. McElin; and B. D. Reeves. "Premenstrual Tension: Symptoms and Weight Changes Related to Potassium Therapy." *American Journal of Obstetrics and Gynecology*, April 1, 1971.

Gruba, Glen H.; and Michael Rohbaugh. "MMPI Correlates of Menstrual Distress." *Psychosomatic Medicine*, 37 (May–June 1975), no. 3.

Haeger, K. "Long-Time Treatment of Intermittent Claudication with Vitamin E." *American Journal of Clinical Nutrition*, 27 (October 1974), no. 10.

Kakulas, Byron A.; and Raymond D. Adams. "Principals of Myopathology as Illustrated in the Nutritional Myopathy of the Rottnes Quokka (Setonix Brachyurus)." *New York Academy of Sciences Annals*, 138 (1969), no. 1.

Kamimura, Mitsuo. "Antiinflammatory Activity of Vitamin E." *The Journal of Vitaminology*, 18 (1972).

Kerr, G. D. "The Management of the Premenstrual Syndrome." *Current Medical Research and Opinion*, 4 (1977), suppl. 4.

Lawrence, J. D.; and H. A. Bern. "Mucous Metaplasia and Mucous Gland Formation in Keratinized Adult Epithelium in SITU Treated with Vitamin A." *Experimental Cell Research*, 21 (1961).

———; R. C. Bower; W. P. Riehl; and J. L. Smith. "Effects of α Tocopherol Acetate on the Swimming Endurance of Trained Swimmers." *The American Journal of Clinical Nutrition*, 28 (March 1975).

Lithgow, D. M.; and W. M. Politzer. "Vitamin A in the Treatment of Menor-
rhagia." *South African Medical Journal,* February 12, 1977.

Little, Betsy Carter; R. J. Matta; and T. P. Zahn. "Physiological and Psychological Effects of Progesterone in Man." *The Journal of Nervous and
Mental Disease,* 159 (1974).

MacDonald, I. "Relationship Between Dietary Carbohydrates and Lipid Me-
tabolism." *Nutrio and Dieta,* 15 (1970).

Parlee, Mary Brown. "Stereotypic Beliefs and Menstruation: A Methodologi-
cal Note on the Moos Menstrual Distress Questionnaire and Some New
Data." *Psychosomatic Medicine,* 36 (May–June 1974), no. 3.

Pellanda, E. B. "Diuretic Action of Estradiol." *Annales d'Endocrinologie,*
Paris, 36 (1975).

Reeves, Billy D.; James E. Garvin; and Thomas W. McElin. "Premenstrual
Tension: Symptoms and Weight Changes Related to Potassium Therapy." *American Journal of Obstetrics and Gynecology,* 109 (April
1971), no. 7.

Reynolds, W. Ann; R. M. Pitkin; A. E. Bauman; G. A. Williams; and G. K.
Hargis. "Calcitonin Secretion in Response to Hypercalcemia in the Fetal
Monkey." *Society for Gynecologic Investigation,* 8 (1977).

Schiff, Isaac, M.D.,; D. Tulchinsky, M.D.; and J. J. Ryan, M.D. "Vaginal
Absorption of Estrone and 17-Estradiol." *Fertility and Sterility,* The
American Fertility Society, 28 (1977), no. 10.

Scutt, Jocelynne A. "A Factor in Female Crime." *Criminology* (1974).

Sesin, George Paul, M.D. "Potassium Chloride Policy." *Pharmacy & Therapeutics Review,* an official publication of the [Boston, Mass.] Beth Is-
rael Hospital Pharmacy & Therapeutics Committee, 1 (1979), no. 3.

Solomon, D.,; D. Strummer; P. P. Nair. "Relationship Between Vitamin E
and Urinary Excretion of Ketosteroid Fractions in Cystic Mastitis." *New
York Academy of Sciences,* Annals 203 (December 1972), no. 18.

Speirs, J.; and R. Jacobson. "The Consumption of Ice as a Symptom of Iron
Deficiency." *South African Medical Journal* 50, October 9, 1976.

Wasserman, R. H.; and A. N. Taylor. "Metabolic Roles of Vitamins D, E,
and K." *Annual Review of Biochemistry,* 41 (1972).

Index

Index